Promotin

an issue for nursing

Other books in the series

Key Management Skills in Nursing Series

Series Editors: Roswyn A Brown
and George Castledine

Promoting Health:
An issue for nursing

Nicola Mackintosh
BSc(Hons), MSc, Dip OHC, RGN

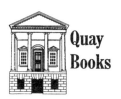

Quay
Books

B. Kilbon

Quay Books, Division of Mark Allen Publishing Limited
Jesses Farm, Snow Hill, Dinton, Nr Salisbury, Wilts, SP3 5HN

©Mark Allen Publishing Ltd, 1996
ISBN 1-85642-094 9

British Library Cataloguing-in-Publication Data
A catalogue record for this book is available from the British
Library

Printed and bound in Great Britain by
Biddles Ltd, Guildford and King's Lynn

Contents

Acknowledgements

A special thanks must go to Louise Wilby, Kate Sanders, Lisa Holcroft and Karyn Noy for their hard work, support and constructive criticism of the draft documents. Similarly, I am indebted to my parents, Patricia and Hugh Mackintosh for their time (which is a precious commodity in their household!), encouragement and helpful feedback. As a team of commentators, they were invaluable and they may have made themselves indispensable for the future!

I am grateful to Roswyn Brown for her ideas and enthusiasm. I always managed to feel inspired when I came away from her house! Thanks also to Kath Butler for managing to turn my ideas into such descriptive cartoons.

But most importantly, I would like to thank Russell for his support. His understanding and patience were my constant source of motivation, without which I could not have finished this book.

Foreword

Nici Mackintosh has produced a benchmark publication which will make a significant contribution to enabling nurses to promote health in an informed and positive way. She examines innovative methods of moving away from the traditionally biomedically oriented behaviour change models of health promotion.

Her suggestions for adopting the Health of the Nation (Department of Health, 1992) in order to incorporate concepts of self-employment, social change and community development are both exciting and realistic. Her analysis powerfully demonstrates the ability of the Master's prepared practitioner to share ideas about exploiting policy challenges and constraints in a way which will benefit us all in the health promotion stakes.

Contrary to the traditional view of professional territorialism in relation to knowledge control, Nici has enhanced the notion of best practice in health promotion by her willingness to share and cascade her ideas and understanding of this important area of nursing practice.

I am sure that, like me, many nurses will be indebted to Nici for demystifying this increasingly significant aspect of both our professional and personal lives as we go forward to the new millennium. Any investment that we make in this direction will be returned a thousand-fold, for, as Izaac Walton (1653) reminds us: '...*health is the second blessing that we mortals are capable of, a blessing that money cannot buy.*'

Walton, I (1653) *The Compleat Angler*

Roswyn Brown
MPhil, BA, RN, RM, DN(London), Cert Ed (Birmingham), RNT, FRSH
Principle Lecturer, Advanced Nursing Practice
Research Unit, Faculty of Health & Social Science
University of Central England in Birmingham

Introduction

*'I keep thinking, here I am about to advise this patient
to stop smoking and to start eating sensibly, when only
10 minutes ago I stuffed a jam doughnut down and had
a quick cigarette myself...*

(Anon)

I suspect that this quote typifies what many nurses believe
health promotion to be. What is health promotion? Does it
involve 'giving advice'? Is it about expecting nurses to act as
role models for health?

There is no doubt that a lot of confusion exists about the
concept and practical application of health promotion. From
my experience as a nurse in practice, and from discussions
with other nurses, midwives and health visitors, I have come
to the conclusion that, as a group of 'health professionals',
most of us are actually ill-equipped to 'promote health'! How
many of us have given out a few leaflets and offered a few
words of advice, and then either mentally ticked off or
documented that we have *done* some health promotion? At
some time or other, how many of us have felt a sense of failure,
when clients have ignored our words of advice and continued
to smoke? How many of us have also felt inadequate when
dealing with a client's complex health needs?

Our general lack of understanding of how to apply health
promotion *in practical terms* is also evident from the research

findings. This is not surprising when it is considered that there used to be little preparation in the general, district nursing, midwifery, health visiting and occupational health nursing syllabi for the knowledge and skills required to undertake this role. Project 2000 and the various diploma and degree courses now have seriously addressed health promotion in their curricula. However, while the generation of new practitioners have benefited from the changes in course content, it seems unrealistic to expect those nurses who received their professional preparation before the advent of the new programmes to take on this role effectively.

In addition, there is the recent surge of interest in health promotion. Suddenly, politicians, the media and the public are all talking about it. 'Health nursing' is now being advocated as the way forward. Jargonistic phrases such as 'self-empowerment' and 'critical consciousness-raising' are being bandied about. Nurses are informed that health professionals need to stop trying to change people's behaviour and must instead equip individuals with life skills. Nurses seem to be swept along by this tide of health promotion fervour, when I suspect that few working in practice stop to think what the terms actually mean, let alone feel comfortable with their practical application.

Despite the fact that the number of textbooks on health promotion is rapidly increasing, there is still a need for a comprehensive, practical guide for nurses which takes into account the specific and varied nature of their work. This book aims to fill this gap and 'demystify' the topic of health promotion for nurses working in practice. It is primarily directed at those who would like to grasp a basic understanding of *how* to promote health from the macro to the micro level, both professionally and personally. However, it should also be of benefit to those with extensive experience, knowledge and skills within the field of health promotion.

Initially, the book sets the scene and discusses health promotion within the context of the public health movement. It raises some of the dilemmas and considers the ethical implications of the different methods of practice. It then focuses on health promotion in nursing and discusses the health strategy *Health of the Nation* (Department of Health, 1992). Finally, a way forward for promoting health in nursing is identified.

The text does not come to a series of conclusions, but is designed to stimulate thought and reflection, thus allowing individual practitioners to choose their own health promotion strategies. It is therefore written as a discussion document with practical examples for illustration. References in the chapters are also kept to a minimum. For those readers who wish to follow up some of the issues mentioned in the text, recommendations for further reading are listed at the end of each chapter. Summary points are used throughout the text to aid the readers to refresh their memories with the main points.

This book is designed to appeal to nurses, midwives and health visitors. It should also benefit and provide interest to lay people and other health-care professionals. It is, however, aimed at those who work with adults. This is not to deny that there is great scope for health action for children and their families, but this needs to be addressed in a separate publication.

While it is acknowledged that nursing, midwifery and health visiting are different professions, each embracing a subtle difference in their philosophy of care, for the purpose of simplicity it has been necessary to use the generic term 'nurse' and 'nursing' in the text. Thus, unless otherwise specified, these terms refer to nurses, midwives and health visitors. However, in some instances mention will be made of one particular discipline.

At times, it has been necessary in the text to distinguish between the nurse and the client. For the sake of clarity, I have chosen to refer to the nurse as 'she' and the client as 'he'. This should not be seen as discriminatory.

This book is designed to enable nurses to recognise their unique role within the multidisciplinary model of health promotion. If it also allows nurses, midwives and health visitors to *value* their contributions as carers and to identify with the values and beliefs that are consistent with promoting health, it will have succeeded.

Nicola Mackintosh:
BSc(Hons), MSc, Dip OHC, RGN
Lecturer in Nursing Studies
Nightingale Institute
King's College
University of London

Chapter 1

Setting the context

This chapter discusses:
- What is 'health'?
- The Public Health Movement
- The New Public Health Movement
- The role of the World Health Organization in health promotion
- Defining health promotion
- Strategies of health education
- Health promotion as a set of values

What is 'health'?

What does the term 'health' actually mean? Is your understanding of health likely to differ from the understanding that a colleague has of the same term? The answer of course is 'yes'. This is because health as a concept is very *personal*. It has a relevance for each and every one of us. Each individual also attaches a *value* to his/her idea of health. These individual beliefs about health arise as a result of the different nature of our life experiences. Therefore, an elderly woman's beliefs about what health means to her are likely to differ from those of a teenage boy.

Thus, although people talk freely about 'feeling healthy' or 'looking healthy', it is important to realise that these statements are left open to interpretation.

So what different perceptions do people hold about health?

Health can be taken to mean:
- a sense of emotional well-being
- happiness
- laughter
- a positive outlook
- emotional energy
- a sense of relaxed calm
- a sense of inner confidence
- a belief in yourself
- possession of life-skills, eg. being assertive
- a certain outward appearance, ie. being slim, pretty, having shining hair
- stamina
- an ability to cope with difficulties
- a sense of physical well-being
- physical fitness and activity
- functioning well at work
- physical energy
- mental energy
- being of use to society
- having the ability to reproduce

However, health is not only perceived in a positive way. Health can also be regarded as an absence of negative factors. In this case, individuals may find it easier to define the concept of ill-health.

Ill-health can be taken to mean:
- lack of physical fitness
- being overweight or underweight
- lacking energy
- being emotionally unstable

- eating all the 'wrong foods'
- working too hard
- being out of control
- being a victim of circumstance
- being unable to cope
- failing to give anything to society

Health in this case is seen as the **absence** of these factors. Similarly, the idea of being ill, sick or in pain may mean more to an individual than the concept of feeling healthy. In this case, a woman may perceive herself as healthy if she has no signs or symptoms of illness.

To summarise, perceptions of health vary; health can be seen in a positive light as having energy and feeling happy, or it can be seen as being synonymous with the absence of negative factors such as illness, pain or unhappiness.

Defining health

The medical model tends to view health as the absence of illness or disease. A medical health assessment is therefore based on determining whether the client has any signs or symptoms of a disease process. If a disease is present, specific medical treatment will then commence to enable the individual to return to health.

In contrast, the focus in nursing theory has been on holistic care rather than on consideration of the individual as a series of unconnected parts. In the same way, health can be seen as a complex concept made up of various dimensions. It is helpful to consider each of these dimensions to build up a picture of exactly how complex the concept of health is. However, it is also important to realise that all these dimensions overlap and interlink.

These dimensions can be broken down into:

health for survival

- food
- water
- shelter
- warmth (heat and clothing)
- peace

health of the emotions

- love
- intimacy
- respect for one another
- a sense of belonging
- companionship
- a sense of fulfilment
- autonomy
- communication

health of the mind

- challenge and fulfilment
- stimulation
- opportunities for development

health of the environment

- safe, clean environment
- safe disposal of waste
- protection of the environment
- environmental opportunities

health of the body

- recreation
- rest

health of the spirit

- sense of belonging
- sense of purpose

Summary:

- health is a multidimensional, holistic concept
- each individual perceives the concept of health differently
- health is not just an absence of illness
- health is a human value

'Health can only be shared. There is no health for me without my brother. There is no health for Britain without Bangladesh' (Wilson, 1975).

The public health movement

The concept of 'public health' developed in response to the mass epidemics of infectious diseases in the 1840s. Industrialisation had resulted in a sudden explosion of urban development and population migration, and a massive increase in the total size of the population. At this time, unemployment, poor working conditions, factory labour, low wages, poor housing and poor health were common among the lower classes. There were epidemics of infectious diseases, primarily cholera, typhus, tuberculosis and smallpox. There was a widespread fear of infection and death.

Inevitably, because of their poor housing and working conditions, disease was more common among the poverty-stricken, working-class population. In contrast, the middle classes had largely benefited from urban development and industrialisation. The middle-class population viewed these epidemics as a sign of a general moral and political decay.

Illness and disease were publicly regarded as:

- directly related to the individual's particular lifestyle
- self-induced
- due to the individual's moral failings

The middle classes became increasingly concerned about the spiralling costs of poor relief. Many regarded the high death rate among the poor as a welcome means of controlling their population size. One who publicly stated his beliefs in the form of an essay on population was the Reverend Thomas Malthus (1798).

In contrast, there were other eminent public figures, principally socialists, who recognised that there was a social cause to the pattern of disease among the poor. A barrister, Edwin Chadwick, saw the need to find and treat the causes of the epidemics in order to restore social order.

In the desire to re-establish some form of social control, alternative theories were suggested to explain the cause of the epidemics. The two main schools of thought were:

- the 'public health' approach
- the 'biomedical' approach

The 'public health' approach

The public health approach arose out of the belief that disease was the result of foul air or 'miasma'. Chadwick was a believer in the miasmata theory. He believed that filth and smells arising from contaminated water had led to the epidemics. He conceived that diseases were spread through water and detailed various sanitary maps in his 'sanitary report' (1842). Chadwick recognised the importance of the environment for public health and argued for clean water, improved drainage and better housing conditions. In 1848 the Public Health Act was passed, which aimed to reduce the spread of water-borne infectious diseases by adequate water supplies and sewerage systems.

Interestingly, the public health movement grew out of a desire to restore social control rather than out of a desire to achieve health for all. While disease was not acknowledged as being directly attributable to poverty, the public health approach did focus on environmental factors.

The biomedical approach

The biomedical approach was initially overshadowed by the public health movement. Medical practitioners largely focused on regarding disease as an imbalance of the bodily fluids. Medical thought often contained a large element of superstition and moral judgment.

Biomedicine started to develop in the 1860s with the advent of medical dissection and medical investigation of paupers. There was the development of 'sanitary reform' and of middle-class female hospital nursing.

In the 1870s, as the focus shifted to the germ theory of disease, the public health movement started to decline. The Contagious Diseases Acts represented the start of authoritarian medical inspection to combat venereal disease. In 1872 and 1875, Public Health Acts were passed to establish sanitary authorities and medical authorities.

The 1870s marked the start of a steady decline in the mortality rate. However, as infant mortality rates remained high, the focus shifted towards the education of families about child health. Lack of parental knowledge about child health was thought to be the problem, rather than poverty or environmental issues. This led to the appointment of health visitors at the end of the 19th century. Community and school nursing were also introduced.

Gradually, in the 1900s, with the development of clean water supplies, better housing, immunisation and other public health measures, the public health movement continued to decline. Emphasis shifted from improving the environment to a focus on the individual with a view to changing individual behaviour patterns.

The 1930s saw the introduction of medical interventions such as sulphonamides and insulin. The death rate which had been steadily falling was reduced further by mass programmes of radiography, vaccination, immunisation and chemotherapy. The conflict that had existed between the medical approach and the public health approach started to disappear as the former became the more dominant. Gradually, resources were shifted from the departments of public health to acute hospital-based services. Similarly, the power of the local authorities was weakened despite them being responsive to the needs of the community. Local authority involvement in health was minimised as they increasingly lost control of hospitals, social workers and community health services (including health visitors and school health services).

Summary:

- the concept of 'public health' arose in the 1840s in response to the crisis caused by the mass epidemics
- the public health movement focused on environmental change and led to improved water supplies and sewage drainage systems
- in the 1870s, the medical approach started to develop with the advent of the germ theory — the focus moved from the environment to the individual
- with the advent of mass immunisations, vaccinations, radiotherapy and chemotherapy in the 1930s, the public health approach disappeared

---

The new public health movement

Today, renewed interest in public health matters has led to the adoption of the term 'the new public health'. This movement could be said to have arisen out of a 20th Century crisis of economic and urban deprivation similar to that which occurred in the 19th century.

The health crisis now

There is:
- poverty
- social class, gender, geographical and racial inequalities in health
- homelessness
- poor housing conditions
- unemployment
- environmental hazards
- environmental pollution by industries and agriculture
- misleading food advertising
- polluted inland water
- polluted sea water
- noise pollution
- traffic pollution
- dangerous disposal systems for waste
- health and safety threats at work
- major disasters

There are also other concerns. Advertising companies continue to promote alcohol and tobacco consumption. Pharmaceutical companies remain the main beneficiaries of research for new treatments. Powerful lobbies exist (eg. the food manufacturing and agricultural lobbies) which have a strong influence over political decision making. Baby milk substitutes are still marketed in most countries in preference to promoting breast feeding, especially in the Third World.

Interestingly, with the rise of the new public health, a similar conflict could arise between the medical approach and the public health movement, as occurred in the 19th century.

What is the new public health?

The new public health aims to reduce poverty and ensure a healthier environment for all. It is concerned with working with local communities to minimise environmental risks and to promote physical, social and economic well-being.

The new public health is:

'...the organised application of resources to achieve the greatest health for the greatest number' (Brotherston, 1991).

The World Health Organization (WHO) has identified the improvement of the health of those living in cities as a priority for public health. The 'Healthy Cities' project was set up to focus health action at the city level, raising public and political awareness. A number of community health projects have also developed involving those at local level. WHO has also developed a 'Health-Promoting Hospital' initiative to reorientate the focus of care in hospitals towards positive health.

Thus, public health action is concerned with working in partnership with many different areas, in *multisectoral collaboration*, involving the public, industry, local government, voluntary organisations, the health service and central government. This will involve providing information, strengthening links between community groups, providing forums for discussions to raise awareness of public health issues, campaigning for equal health rights for all individuals, promoting research and evaluation, and developing policies for health. Public health is an important resource that needs nourishing and valuing by us all.

The role of the WHO in health promotion

The WHO was created in 1948. As its name suggests, it is primarily concerned with world health problems. It has always tried to be apolitical, which of course has proved difficult as most health issues in reality have some form of political agenda.

WHO's first important document outlining the way forward for health promotion was the Alma Ata declaration in 1977 (WHO, 1978). This declaration identified its main target as the improvement of health and health-related problems for all, by the year 2000, known today as *Health For All 2000*.

Health For All 2000 *has six main themes:*

- equity — achieving fairness by targeting inequalities in health
- health promotion — promoting a positive sense of health
- community participation — letting those at the grass roots level participate in decision making
- multisectoral cooperation — involving all the public and private sectors
- primary health care — providing locally defined services to the community at large
- international cooperation — working with other countries to address global problems such as pollution, deforestation and the exploitation of Third World countries

As it was anticipated that difficulties would arise as a result of putting such a far reaching strategy as this into practice, certain targets were drawn up by WHO. The aim of these was to aid the application and evaluation of *Health For All 2000* (WHO, 1985).

Health For All 2000 *targets:*

- the first group of targets looks at how to reduce the inequalities that exist between different countries and between different groups of people
- the second group looks at promoting healthy lifestyles, healthy behaviour and environmental health, not only on an individual basis, but also on a structural basis (eg. changing policies)

- the third group outlines the necessary systems that are needed to support the above actions (eg. research, information networks and educational programmes)

The next stage was to draw up an action plan. A health promotion action plan was devised and named the *Ottawa Charter* (WHO, 1986).

Ottawa Charter *for health promotion action:*

- to make health everyone's responsibility, not just the responsibility of those working in the health service, to put health on the agenda of policy makers at all levels, to use a variety of approaches (eg. legislation and organisational change) in order to make the healthy choice the easy choice
- to conserve the natural environment, to care for one another on a local, national and world basis, to enable the creation of a healthy society where living and working conditions have a positive impact on health
- to develop community involvement in health issues, to encourage self-help programmes, to develop public participation in health action
- to develop personal and social development through the provision of education, information and social skills
- to extend the role of the health sector beyond the curative to the promotion of health, to reorientate the service to one that is sensitive to the individual's needs

So what skills do people need to promote the sort of health action outlined in the *Ottawa Charter*? The *Charter* outlines three important process methodologies, or three ways *how* to implement health promotion action.

The 'how' of health promotion action:

- by advocacy — fighting for health issues, putting health on the agenda
- by enablement — giving someone the authority or expertise to take control
- by mediation — working together with others, acting as a go-between

Defining health promotion

WHO has provided us with an authorised view of health promotion which is now widely accepted (WHO, 1984). It is important to be aware, however, that it is a 'global' view, taken from a body primarily concerned with global issues of health. Others have attempted therefore to define the main features of health promotion at a more local level. This has been no easy task and has led to much confusion and contradiction.

A working definition of health promotion

Prior to the 1980s, the term widely used was 'health education'. Several attempts had been made to break down the various approaches incorporated in health education. There was disagreement about the aims and objectives of education for health. Was the aim to bring about a change in an individual's behaviour or was it purely to give information, allowing the individual the freedom to choose a pattern of behaviour?

To complicate matters, in the 1980s the new term 'health promotion' emerged. Where did health education fit in the picture of health promotion? Was health promotion just a glossy new name for what was essentially the same practice as health education? It was a time of much confusion and argument.

Finally, the majority of authors came to the conclusion that the two terms are different, and health education is only one part of health promotion. Health promotion in its broadest sense can therefore be classed as any activity that fosters health.

Health promotion can cover:
- activities designed to encourage well-being and positive health
- use of the mass media in awareness raising
- community programmes and self-help groups

- development of policies at local and national level
- campaigns, either on the national or local level
- immunisation programmes
- the activities of powerful lobbies
- health education

Health promotion usually refers to activities on a large scale. It involves social, economic and political change in order to ensure that the environment is conducive to health. Health promotion not only encompasses a nurse educating an individual about his health needs, but also demands that the nurse plays her part in attempting to address the wider environmental and social issues that adversely affect people's health.

Health education, as a part of health promotion, usually refers to those activities which raise an individual's awareness, giving the individual the health knowledge required to enable him to decide on a particular health action.

The two terms can be defined as follows:

*'**Health promotion** covers all aspects of those activities that seek to improve the health status of individuals and communities. It therefore includes both health education and all attempts to produce environmental and legislative change conducive to good health'* (Dennis *et al*, 1982).

*'**Health education** is concerned with raising individuals' competence and knowledge about health and illness, about the body and its functions, about prevention and coping; with raising competence and knowledge to use the health-care system and to understand its functions; and with raising awareness about social, political and environmental factors that influence health'* (Baric, 1985).

Summary:

- health promotion and health education are not interchangeable terms
- health education is on a smaller scale and usually targets the individual or groups of people
- health promotion is on a large scale and involves targeting the environment, or the political or social structure, both nationally and internationally
- health education is only a small part of health promotion

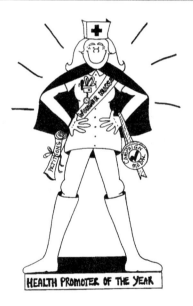

HEALTH PROMOTER OF THE YEAR

Strategies of health education

Just to confuse matters further, the term 'health education' can also be broken down into various different approaches. Many authors have tried to classify these approaches. I have looked at five of the commonly identified approaches and compared their different practical applications and goals:

Behaviour change approach

- focus — the individual
- goal — to persuade the individual to adopt a particular lifestyle or listen to medical advice, to prevent or limit disease and reduce mortality/morbidity rates
- rationale — curative medicine cannot cope with current rate of disease. Prevention is better/cheaper than cure
- evaluation — measured on whether or not the individual adopts a particular lifestyle or changes his behaviour

eg. advising/persuading the individual to give up smoking

Educational approach

- focus — the individual
- goal — to help the individual develop his knowledge and skills, to help him explore his attitudes, so that he can make an informed choice about his health
- rationale — education is about freedom of choice
- evaluation — measured on the facilitation of decision making, irrespective of the nature of the decision actually made

eg. presenting the individual with the facts about smoking and leaving him to make a choice

Social change approach

- focus — the physical and social environment
- goal — to make healthy choices the easy choices by changing the physical and social environment. Also aims to raise individuals' awareness and involvement in health issues in order to stimulate the demand for social change
- rationale — the root of health problems lies in social, economic and political factors
- evaluation — measured by the implementation of social, political or environmental change

eg. campaigning for smoke-free areas, lobbying parliament for an advertising ban on tobacco

Self-empowerment (humanistic) approach

- focus — the individual
- goal — to facilitate decision making by improving how the individual feels about himself
- rationale — by developing motivation, self-confidence and life skills the individual is in a better position to identify his own health needs and take action to meet them
- evaluation — measured by the development of decision-making skills and life skills

eg. enabling the individual to identify why he smokes, helping the individual to develop the confidence and skills needed for him to make a choice and implement his own health plan

Community development approach

- focus — a group
- goal — to help a group work together, find their common interests and fight their particular health cause
- rationale — it is better to work from the group's valuable experiences rather than to work from a professionally defined agenda
- evaluation — measured by successful public awareness raising of the group's concerns and the implementation of health action for the benefit of the group

eg. identifying a need for a self-help group, facilitating the group, acting as resource and supporter for the group

Health promotion as a set of values

These approaches help to illustrate the principles of health education in practice. However, classifications of this sort can also lead to an oversimplification of the concept of health education. Similarly, there is a danger that the act of boxing and categorising health promotion ensures that its very essence is lost.

Health promotion (and health education as part of it) is more than a set of activities. It is a term that embodies a set of values and beliefs. It is about an outlook, a conviction and a code of conduct which affects the way relationships are created. Promoting health means putting health not only on people's personal agenda, but also on the public agenda so that it becomes an integral part of everyone's way of life.

Examples of these five health education approaches have been consistently used in the chapters as a simple guide to illustrate the issues involved. However, the theme of health promotion as a set of values also runs throughout the book. This theme is also examined in detail in chapter six.

Summary:

- health education can take the form of any of five approaches; behaviour change, educational, social change, self-empowerment and community development
- while examination of these approaches helps to illustrate the practical application of health education, there is a danger that the essence of health education and health promotion are lost
- health promotion is about a set of values

References

Baric L (1985) The meaning of words: health promotion. *J Inst Health Educ* **23**(1): 367–72

Brotherston J (1991) A public health approach. In: Draper P, ed. *Health Through Public Policy: The Greening of Public Health*. Green Print, London

Chadwick E (1842) *Report from the Poor Law Commissioners on an inquiry into the Sanitary Condition of the labouring population of Great Britain*. HMSO, London

Dennis J, Draper P, Holland S, Snipster P, Speller V, Sunter J *et al* (1982) *Health promotion in the reorganised NHS*. The Health Services, 26 Nov

Malthus T (1798) An essay on the principle of population. In: Draper P, ed. *Health Through Public Policy: The Greening of Public Health*. Green Print, London

Wilson M (1975) *Health is for People*. Longman and Todd, Darton

World Health Organization (1978) *Primary Health Care*. Report on the International Conference on Primary Health Care. Alma Ata 1977, WHO/UNICEF, USSR, Geneva

World Health Organization (1984) *Health Promotion: A Discussion Document on the Concepts and Principles*. WHO, Copenhagen

World Health Organization (1985) *Targets For Health For All. Targets in Support of the European Regional Strategy for Health For All*. WHO, Regional Office for Europe, Copenhagen

World Health Organization (1986) *Ottawa Charter for Health For All. An International Conference on Health Promotion*. WHO, Geneva

Further reading

Health

Aggleton P (1991) *Health*. Routledge, London
- An introduction to the sociology of health. This book raises important issues and provides debate about explanations for patterns of health

Baelz PR (1979) Philosophy of health education. In: Sutherland I ed, *Health Education: Perspectives and Choices*, 1st edn. Allen and Unwin, London: 20–39
- This chapter explores the values and beliefs that underpin the concept of health

Cribb A, Dines A (1993) What is health? In: Dines A, Cribb A eds, *Health Promotion: concepts and practice*. Blackwell Scientific, Oxford: 3–19
- This first chapter discusses the definition and meaning of the term health

Ewles L, Simnett I (1992) *Promoting Health: A Practical Guide*, 2nd edn. Scutari, London
- Chapter one provides a simple guide to the key concepts of health

Naidoo J, Wills J (1994) *Health Promotion: Foundations for Practice*. Bailliere Tindall, London
- Chapter one explores the concept of health

Seedhouse D (1986) *Health: Foundations for Achievement*. John Wiley & Sons, Chichester
- This book provides a comprehensive, theoretical discussion about the meaning and sense of the word 'health'

Public health

Ashton J, Seymour H (1988) *The New Public Health*. Open University Press, Milton Keynes
- This book traces the historical development of public health

Draper P (1991) A public health approach. In: Draper P ed, Health Through Public Policy: The Greening of Public Health. Green Print, London: 7–25
- Chapter one explores the origins of public health and discusses public policy

Hogg C (1991) *Healthy Change: Towards Equality in Health*. Socialist Health Association, London
- Chapter one looks at environmental and public health

Macdonald G, Bunton R (1992) Health promotion: discipline or disciplines? In: Bunton R Macdonald G (eds) *Health Promotion: Disciplines and Diversity*. Routledge, London
- Chapter one puts health promotion in a public health context

Sutherland I (1979) History and background. In: Sutherland I ed. *Health Education: Perspectives and Choices*, 1st edn. Allen and Unwin, London: 1–18
- Chapter one details the history of public health

World Health Organization

Tones BK (1986) Health education and the ideology of health promotion: a review of alternative approaches. *Health Educ Res* **1**(1): 3–12

Tones BK (1990) Positive health. *Nursing* **4**: 22
- These two articles explore the role of the World Health Organization in health promotion

Definition and strategies of health promotion

Baric L (1985) The meaning of words: health promotion. *J Inst Health Educ* **23**(1): 367–72
- This article discusses the difference in meaning between the two terms health education and health promotion

Beattie A (1991) Knowledge and control in health promotion: a test case for social policy and social theory. In: Gabe J, Calnan M, Bury M, eds, *The Sociology of The Health Service.* Routledge, London: 162–202
- This chapter details the author's own structural map of health promotion

Cribb A, Dines A (1993) What is health promotion? In: Dines A, Cribb A, eds, *Health Promotion: concepts and practice.* Blackwell Scientific, Oxford: 20–33
- This chapter provides a detailed theoretical discussion of the difference in meaning between the terms health education and health promotion

Downie RS, Fyfe C, Tannahill A (1990) *Health Promotion: Models and Values.* Oxford Medical Publications, Oxford
- These authors classify seven domains of health promotion

Ewles L, Simnett I (1992) *Promoting Health: A Practical Guide*, 2nd edn. Scutari, London
- Chapter two discusses definitions and a framework for health promotion activities. Chapter three details models of health education

French J, Adams L (1986) From analysis to synthesis: Theories of health education. *Health Educ J* **45**(2): 71–4
- The authors propose a triphasic model of health education

Naidoo J, Wills J (1994) '*Health Promotion: Foundations for Practice*'. Bailliere Tindall, London
- Chapter five provides a thorough description of the different types of approach to health promotion

Tones BK (1985) Health promotion — a new panacea? *J Inst Health Educ* **23**: 16–21
- The article discusses the term health promotion and the ways it has been used

Tones BK (1986) Health education and the ideology of health promotion: a review of alternative approaches. *Health Educ Res* **1**(1): 3–12
- The author proposes three major emphases to health education

World Health Organization (1984) *Health Promotion: A Discussion Document on the Concepts and Principles*. WHO, Copenhagen
- This document presents a summary of the working group

Chapter 2

Dilemmas in health promotion

Having given a general picture of health promotion, we can now look at some of the important issues that surround the concept and practice of health promotion.

This chapter discusses:

- Responsibility for health
- The determinants of health
- The politics of health
- The targeting of resources

Responsibility for health

Where does the responsibility for health actually lie?

- should individuals be held responsible for the outcomes of their health actions?

or

- is it unfair to hold individuals responsible, as in reality they are often constrained by factors outside their control?

There is a particular school of thought that believes that people are able to accept or reject social pressures and are therefore free to choose and decide for themselves. Members of this group are known as 'existentialists' and they believe that the responsibility for health lies firmly with the individual. In the existentialist's opinion, the individual has the choice to accept or reject a particular course of health action and thus can be directly blamed if the action results in a breakdown of health.

In contrast, others believe that although people may perceive themselves as free, in reality their behaviour is determined by other forces. These people are known as 'determinists' and they argue that individuals are products of the environment, and factors such as race, gender, social class and genetics are the actual determinants of health. The determinist believes that the individual cannot therefore be held responsible for a health action.

Although agreeing with certain aspects of both existentialism and determinism, it is too straightforward to assume that either the individual has freedom of choice over his health or that the individual's health is predetermined. Perhaps the way forward is to develop a more eclectic approach and use certain elements from both of these rationales to underpin an analysis and understanding about health promotion.

Health circles of influence

To explore this issue further, the many factors that influence health need to be considered. It is apparent that while some of these factors appear to be within an individual's control, there are others over which the individual seems to have little influence.

There are some factors that affect health that may, in some situations, be within an individual's control, yet in different circumstances be outside it. For example, a parent may be limited to choosing a school within a certain radius of home, but may still have a choice of three schools to pick from. Similarly, an individual may have a choice of whether to extend her responsibilities at work, which is likely to be associated with increased stress. She may also be under a lot of stress due to the illness of her mother, over which she has little control.

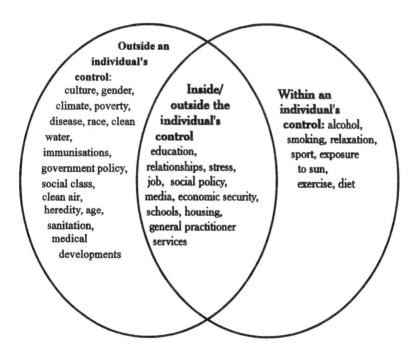

Outside an individual's control: culture, gender, climate, poverty, disease, race, clean water, immunisations, government policy, social class, clean air, heredity, age, sanitation, medical developments

Inside/ outside the individual's control education, relationships, stress, job, social policy, media, economic security, schools, housing, general practitioner services

Within an individual's control: alcohol, smoking, relaxation, sport, exposure to sun, exercise, diet

So how do the existentialist and the determinist make sense of these circles of influence? Obviously, for the existentialist, those influences that are readily identifiable as being within an individual's control, such as smoking and taking exercise, can be used to illustrate the belief that the individual should face the consequences of that behaviour. However, what of those influences that the individual has no control over, such as gender? After all, there is research to show that gender inequalities exist in health. The existentialist claims that people create themselves by means of their decisions and choices. In other words, the existentialist believes that women have a higher morbidity rate than men because they choose to consult their general practitioners (GPs) more frequently than men, and because they choose to acknowledge their feelings of illness more then men.

In contrast, the determinist perceives the individual as having little control over any of the factors influencing health. Social class and gender are obvious examples of factors that determinists believe are beyond the individual's power to change. Thus, determinists believe that social class inequalities in health are caused by factors such as poverty and housing which are beyond the capacity of the individual to alter. In the same way, the determinist perceives gender inequalities as the product of reproductive make-up. In addition, determinists also look to causal explanations other than individual choice to explain why a person smokes, avoids exercise or overeats. They suggest that factors such as unemployment, poverty, peer pressure or cultural norms are to blame for these particular behaviours.

While it is difficult to accept that freedom of choice exists in health matters, the individual does have some control over his behaviour. Removing responsibility for health from the individual denies the person the ability to be autonomous or to self-care. However, factors such as poverty, gender and social class also need to be taken into account as they influence an individual's health action in a way that the individual may be powerless to change.

The opposing views of the existentialist and the determinist have been used to illustrate that, when it comes to people's beliefs about the amount of influence they have over their health, there is much scope for diversity of opinion. There is no easy answer to the question of who should take responsibility for health.

Summary:

- there are many factors that can have an influence on an individual's health
- an individual may be able to control some of these factors, but may be powerless to control others
- opinions differ as to whether the behaviour of an individual is predetermined or whether the individual is free to choose a way of life
- opinions will also differ in determining the level of responsibility the individual should take for health

The determinants of health

In chapter one, the dimensions of health were broken down into the following groups:

- health for survival
- health of the emotions
- health of the mind
- health of the environment
- health of the body
- health of the spirit

In an ideal world, each and every individual should have an equal right to enjoy each of these dimensions of health. The extent to which they experience such factors as 'intimacy' and 'respect for one another' is largely due to the circumstances. However, from an examination of other aspects such as 'food', 'warmth' and 'opportunities for development' it is apparent that certain groups are in a better position to enjoy these than others.

Health for survival:

- food — in the developing countries, not everyone has enough food to survive; in this country, not everyone has the same access to or can afford to buy fresh fruit and vegetables

- warmth — the homeless often do not have access to heat and clothing; some people have problems paying their heating bills
- peace — some groups are more prone to discrimination and verbal/physical abuse; women can be the victims of harassment or rape

Health of the mind:

- opportunities for development — in many Third World countries, people do not have access to education; in this country, not everyone has the same opportunities to develop their education, career or interests

Health of the environment:

- safe, clean environment — the environment is often affected by pollution and waste; in this country, there are many homeless people

These are only a few examples of where inequalities in health status exist between different groups of people and between different populations. By focusing on the inequalities that exist in this country, a pattern emerges of certain factors that are associated with the groups who consistently suffer more ill-health or die prematurely:

- *social class* — those in the lower social classes have higher death rates and experience more illness than those in the higher classes; the former group are also more likely to have lower birth weight babies than those in the higher social classes
- *poverty* —: those on low incomes who are deprived of material comforts are more likely to become ill or die prematurely than those on high incomes
- *housing* — factors such as overcrowding, poor housing conditions and homelessness are all associated with ill health
- *employment* — those out of work are more likely to suffer from ill health than those in employment
- *gender* — women suffer more ill health than men while men die earlier than women

- *ethnic minorities* — the Afro-Caribbean population have a higher incidence of stroke and high blood pressure than the other ethnic groups
- *geographical area* — those living in the north are more likely to die prematurely than those living in the south of England

So how can these inequalities be accounted for? Firstly, it is worth attempting to explain the existence of inequalities in health between the social classes.

The artefact explanation

This explanation suggests that those statistics that show there is a widening gap in mortality between the social classes are actually questionable. This is because the criteria for measuring the social classes has changed over time so that comparisons based on health and class are meaningless. *However, a similar pattern of inequality in health is found if other measures of material advantage, such as education and access to a car, are used instead of social class.*

The selection explanation

Alternatively, this argument suggests that the social class structure is a form of health filter. In other words, a person's health determines his/her social class rather than vice versa. Those in good health move up through the social classes while those with higher levels of illness drift down the social scale. *However, there is little evidence to support this argument.*

Cultural/ behavioural explanation

This third explanation proposes that certain behaviours are associated with the social patterns of ill health. Thus, harmful behaviours such as excess drinking, smoking and eating are more common among the lower social classes. There are also cultural differences between the social groups in their attitudes towards health. The middle class believe that they have control over their way of life, while the working class have a more fatalistic view of health. Those in the lower classes lack the education, or are too reckless or lazy to change their lives. *However, many behaviour patterns, such as smoking and alcohol abuse, are used by the working classes to enable them to cope with the stress of their situation.*

Material/structural explanation

Lastly, this argument suggests that the distribution of health in the population is linked to the distribution of wealth in society. Poverty is seen to have a direct influence on ill health. The reason why the lower social classes experience more ill health is that they have lower incomes, lower levels of education and fewer resources. *Based on the evidence this seems the most plausible explanation.*

If the patterns of ill health within the social classes can largely be accounted for by the unequal distribution of resources in society, can this explanation be used to account for other types of health inequality?

It can be shown that:

- *poverty* is closely linked to the lower social classes
- those on low incomes are also more likely to be *homeless* or live in overcrowded housing
- poverty is associated with *unemployment*; manual labour is often associated with occupational health risks
- *women* are especially vulnerable to poverty; women earn less than men in terms of pay and occupational benefits
- poor health of the *ethnic minorities* is often associated with low income, poor working conditions and poor housing
- the *geographical* differences in health can be partly explained by social class distribution

However, while the importance of material disadvantage needs to be acknowledged, structural explanations cannot account for all the health inequalities that exist between certain groups. Consider the following:

- *certain occupations associated with the higher income groups* may be associated with high levels of stress related illness
- *women of all income groups* suffer more ill health as a result of the stress of the roles enforced upon them by society
- *women of all income groups* are protected from early mortality from coronary heart disease due to the protective action of oestrogen
- *in general, men* suffer higher rates of suicide and accidents than women
- *certain ethnic minority groups* may be discriminated against both in gaining access to health care and during their treatment
- there are *regional variations* within the north–south divide

---

Summary:

- inequalities in health status exist between different groups of people and between different populations
- in this country, inequalities in health can be classed according to social class, gender, race and geography
- patterns of ill health within such groups can largely be explained by an unequal distribution of resources in society

---

The politics of health

Accepting that these inequalities are indeed attributed largely to material disadvantage, then the responsibility for health can be seen to lie not with the individual, but primarily with the State. Addressing these inequalities would have to take the form of social policy changes such as welfare benefits, improved housing and better working conditions.

However, the responsibility for health can also be seen to be 'pluralistic'. In other words, there are a number of other groups who can be viewed as having a part to play in influencing health. While these groups have some responsibility for health, there must also be involvement and commitment to health from decision makers.

Those groups with a responsibility towards health:
- politicians
- economists
- industrialists
- educationalists
- voluntary agencies
- the media
- health service employees

In the last 6 years there have been a number of reforms that have affected service provision in the National Health Service (NHS). These include the introduction of GP contracts, The White Paper *Working for Patients* (Department of Health, 1989a) and the Community Care Act (Department of Health, 1989b). The key change has been the introduction of an internal market within the NHS in which responsibility for purchasing services has been separated from the responsibility for providing them.

Purchasers:
- district health authorities
- GP fundholders

Providers:

- NHS trusts
- directly managed hospitals
- community health services
- integrated hospital and community service trusts
- mental health service trusts
- general practices
- private hospitals

These reforms have had far-reaching implications for health promotion:

- responsibility for the services has been devolved from region to NHS trust hospitals and districts
- the district health authority now has the authority to prioritise health promotion and community services
- responsibility for individual health has been devolved to the individual
- responsibility for the environment has been devolved to local authorities
- directors of public health now have the role of assessing the needs of the population

But:

- the Government still sets national and local targets, effectively constraining providers in some aspects of decision making
- cash restraints often mean that curative services still take priority over health promotion services
- some aspects of health promotion practice, such as community health projects, do not fit easily in the present structure — they would be better located outside the purchaser/provider split
- health education units/health promotion units are part of the district health authority. They may be directly accountable to the Department of Public Health

The delegation of responsibility to local level was aimed at enabling the public to have more of a say in their health care. The reforms were intended to give patients better health care and greater choice of the services available, wherever they lived in the country. It was also hoped that those working within the NHS would gain greater satisfaction and rewards by responding to the local needs of the public.

However, the effects of these reforms have been somewhat different.

Changes resulting from the purchaser/provider split:

- greater choice for the patient. *But patients are still dependent on the district managers and GP fundholders to define their needs. Patients may also have to travel to a hospital which is cheaper rather than to one of their choice*

- better health care for the patient; there has been an increase in the number of outreach clinics, community hospitals and GP surgeries that carry out minor surgery; purchasers are keen to ensure that patients receive a continuous package of care that starts in the community and follows the patient through into the acute sector and back into the community again

- making the service more responsive to the patients needs. *But the fact that the money follows the patient across district boundaries encourages the growth of large specialised hospitals which may be more interested in attracting patients from out of the area than being responsive to local needs*

- multisectoral collaboration; once all the acute and community units have gained trust status, the districts will no longer have responsibility for providing health care, but instead will have responsibility for setting standards and ensuring that multisectoral collaboration occurs. *But to some extent the targets set are dependant on the politics and personalities of the purchasers and foster competition rather than collaborative working*

- reduction in hospital waiting lists. *But while the numbers of patients waiting for long periods has dropped; this has often been at the expense of those waiting for shorter times*
- improvement in quality of care; introduction of medical audit, employment of additional consultants, better communication between provider and purchaser, use of contracts to set standards. *But the essence of high-quality care is often difficult to measure and justify in an environment where the current focus is on the cost of health care and on ensuring that purchasers get 'value for money'*

In addition to the NHS reforms, the White Paper *Promoting Better Health* (Department of Health, 1987) has changed perceptions about health promotion and primary care. This document aimed to emphasise health promotion and disease prevention and to offer more choice and information to patients.

The key changes were:

- to contract GPs to provide regular health checks for all on their list
- to give GPs financial rewards for meeting immunisation targets
- to encourage GPs to take on the role of teaching people how to improve their health
- to devolve ultimate responsibility to the individual for the improvement and maintainance of his/her own health

However, the contract solely focused on the GP and did not incorporate the work of the health visitor or practice nurse.

It was inevitable, though, that the role of the practice nurse did develop in response to the new contract, particularly in relation to health promotion. It is also likely that the role of the practice nurse and health visitor will develop further to take on additional health education responsibilities.

The *Health of the Nation* (Department of Health, 1992) is the first health strategy that has been devised for England. Similar strategies have also been devised for Scotland, Wales and Northern Ireland. The *Health of the Nation* recognises, at least in part, the positive effect on health that social and public health measures have brought about. It therefore calls for everyone to take a part in helping to improve health, and devolves responsibility for health to:

- local government
- the health education authority
- the media
- voluntary organisations
- workplaces
- individuals

But the Government also ensures that it retains ultimate control over setting targets and allocating resources.

By placing emphasis on the promotion of health by changing structures through public policy change and creating healthy surroundings, the White Paper attempts to follow some of the WHO's *Health For All by the Year 2000* Charter (WHO, 1986). Influences on health such as poverty, housing and unemployment are also acknowledged as important.

However, much of the *Health of the Nation* focuses on the prevention rather than the promotion of health and places responsibility on individuals for their own health. More importantly, although structural influences have been acknowledged, little action has actually been taken to address these issues. For example:

- the UK does not meet European community standards in water supplies and for the maintenance of pollutant-free coastal waters suitable for sea bathing
- tobacco is still actively promoted, despite the evidence from other countries of the positive effect of banning tobacco advertising

- the Government actively encourages farmers to produce meat products that are high in fat
- commercial companies spend more money on advertising bottled milk than the Government spends on the promotion of breast feeding, despite the widely acknowledged health benefits of breast milk and the implications of this for the developing countries

All the reforms have been prompted to a certain extent by a discrepancy arising between the money allocated by the Government for the NHS, and the funding needed to meet increasing demand. Although lip service has been paid to the political, social and economic determinants of health, there is little evidence of any major changes in Government policy to address the inequalities that exist in health.

Thus it appears that the White Paper actually ignores the main drive of *Health for All 2000*, which is to reduce inequalities. It hands the responsibility over to the people, but does not equip them with the resources necessary for people to improve their health status. *Health For All 2000* argues for relocating the management of health outside the health service. In contrast, the *Health of the Nation* looks to health professionals to implement a major part of its strategies.

If the majority of health inequalities are due to material disadvantage, then it can be seen that an uneasy relationship exists between wealth and health. Activities are frequently prioritised for their economic value and little regard is paid to their harmful health consequences. Current economic policy seems openly to value wealth more than health. For example, the economic value of tobacco advertising is perceived to outweigh its health damaging effects.

Summary:

- in the last few years, there have been a number of government reforms that have affected the provision of services for the promotion of people's health
- the idea of the purchaser/provider split in health care was to increase choice and the quality of the service for the patient or client; however, the current focus on 'value for money' has often meant that patients or clients have less choice and the service is not individualised to their health needs
- the *Health of the Nation* largely places responsibility for health on the individual; to date there has been little evidence of any Government policies to address structural influences (such as poverty and housing) on health
- current economic policy appears to openly value wealth above health

The targeting of resources

How should money for health be spent?

- is every individual entitled to have the same amount of money spent on his health?

or

- should the money be spent on ensuring that health is afforded to the majority of the population?

The first viewpoint argues for the importance of each and every human life. It suggests that people have the right to choose how to live and that individuals are free to take whatever health action they so wish. This of course means that a person's right to smoke or refuse treatment is respected. Rationing resources takes the form of spreading money spent on health out thinly but equally among all individuals however they choose to live their lives.

If, however, the second viewpoint is adopted, it argues that it is better to risk depriving one individual of his right to choose, if this ensures that greater benefit is afforded to the majority of people. It suggests that a person's rights should not stand in the way of the good of the people. Resources are therefore targeted at protecting the health of the majority of the population even if this adversely affects the health of a few.

There have been numerous programmes of Government intervention implemented to protect the health of the majority of the population. For example:

- smoking bans on public transport
- the fluoridation of water
- compulsory vaccinations
- smoke-free areas in public places

These interventions mean that certain individuals may be forced to take a health action against their wishes, for example refraining from smoking on public transport for the good of the other passengers.

The Government also selects some priorities for health spending. This means targeting resources at certain groups. Although on the positive side this implies that a specific population with a health problem may be the focus of extra resources, there are other implications too:

- by identifying this specific population it may become the focus of unwelcome attention and be stigmatised
- a minority group may be left out or discriminated against

Targeting of resources:

- resources may be restricted to certain groups, eg. coronary artery bypass graft surgery has been limited in some hospitals to non-smokers
- certain groups have greater access to resources, eg. in *Health of the Nation*, teenagers are singled out for health education in order to reduce their pregnancy rates

Summary:

- it is necessary to target and prioritise spending on health as the demand for health care increases
- resources can either be shared equally between all individuals (eg. the principle behind the NHS), or resources can be spent on protecting the health of the majority at the expense of a possible minority
- resources are also targeted at certain groups who have been defined as having a particular health need

References

Department of Health (1989a) *Working for Patients*. White Paper. HMSO, London

Department of Health (1989b) *Caring for People: Community Care in the Next Decade and Beyond*. HMSO, London

Department of Health (1987) *Promoting Better Health*. White Paper. HMSO, London

Department of Health (1992) *The Health of The Nation: A Strategy for Health in England*. HMSO, London

World Health Organization (1986) *Ottawa Charter for Health For All. An International Conference on Health Promotion*. WHO, Geneva

Further reading

Responsibility for health

Jacob F (1994) Ethics in health promotion: freedom or determinism. *Br J Nurs* **3**(6): 299–302

- This article explores nurses' beliefs about human nature and the influence that these beliefs have on their approach to the promotion of health

Determinants of health

Aggleton P (1991) *Health*. Routledge, London
- This book raises important issues and provides debate about explanations for patterns of health

Davey Smith G, Bartley M, Blane D (1990) The Black Report on socio-economic inequalities in health 10 years on. *Br Med J* **301**: 373–5
- This report presents an update since the Black Report was published, and comments that there are persistent and in some cases widening inequalities in health

Hogg C (1991) *Healthy Change*. Socialist Health Association, London
- Chapter four discusses inequalities in health

Jacobson B, Smith A, Whitehead M (1991) *The Nation's Health: A Strategy for the 1990s*. A report from an independant multidisciplinary committee, 2nd edn. King Edward's Hospital Fund for London, London
- This book details statistical material about health trends and discusses responsibilities for health. It also discusses a public health strategy for the 1990s

Naidoo J, Wills J (1994) *Health Promotion: Foundations for Practice*. Bailliere Tindall, London
- Chapter two discusses influences on health

Townsend P, Davidson N, Whitehead M (1992) *Inequalities in Health*, 2nd edn. Penguin, London
- This book combines the Black Report and a review of more recent studies on inequality in health

The politics of health

Draper P (1991) *Health through Public Policy: the Greening of Public Health*. Green Print, London
- This book links health policy to economic factors and discusses the greening of public health

Hogg C (1991) *Healthy Change*. Socialist Health Association, London
- This book provides comprehensive details of a radical reorganisation of public services to enable health for all

Naidoo J, Wills J (1994) *Health Promotion: Foundations for Practice*. Bailliere Tindall, London
- Chapter seven considers the important relationship between health promotion and politics. It also details different political ideologies

Robinson R, LeGrand J, eds (1993) *Evaluating the NHS Reforms*. King's Fund Institute, Policy Journals, London
- This book provides a comprehensive review of the effects of the NHS reforms

Rodmell S, Watt A, eds (1986) *The Politics of Health Education: Raising the Issues*. Routledge and Kegan Paul, London
- This book offers examples of alternative social action strategies to promote health

Chapter 3

Ethical issues in health promotion

So far the concept of health and health promotion have been examined. The dilemmas surrounding the concept and practice of health promotion have also been discussed. In this chapter, the ethical implications of health promotion practice will be addressed. The five health education approaches or strategies will be used as a framework. These are:

- behaviour change
- educational
- social change
- self-empowerment
- community development

Each of these has been considered in turn in order to locate health education within an ethical framework.

This chapter looks at the following:
- Ethical principles
- The ethical implications of each approach

Ethical principles

There are four widely accepted ethical principles (Beauchamp and Childress, 1989):

- respecting an individual's right to not only make his own decisions, but also to act on these decisions as the individual sees fit (autonomy)
- doing good (beneficience)
- doing no harm (non-maleficience)
- being fair and equitable (justice)

If all interactions and activities are guided by these principles in everyday life, then people are more likely to be treated fairly, and harm could be avoided. However, nurses are also likely to encounter ethical conflicts due to the nature of their job. In other words, caring for individuals involves taking decisions and actions that will have an influence on the health of the individual.

Obviously the process of promoting health covers a wide diversity of actions. It can involve selling health messages or trying to influence people's actions. In the previous chapters health promotion was also seen to involve the implementation of Government policies for the good of the majority of people.

The ethical implications of each approach

How does each approach fit into the ethical framework outlined above? The easiest way to discuss this is to look at each strategy in turn.

Behaviour change approach

This approach is based upon the belief that individuals should be held responsible for their health actions. The approach is characteristically used in public campaigns (eg.

national no smoking day) or as methods of persuasion on a one-to-one basis. This is the approach adopted by the Government in *Health of the Nation*. It is also the preferred method adopted by the medical profession.

The health professional perceives herself as the expert. The health professional is seen as having the right to offer professional advice to the client. An assumption is made that, once the health information has been given, the individual will automatically want to comply with the health professional's advice and thus be motivated to change his behaviour.

So if the behaviour change approach is adopted, how do the methods measure up against each of the ethical principles noted above?

Respect for an individual's right to self-rule

In the process of trying to change an individual's behaviour, health information is shared with the individual. This raises the individual's health awareness and enables the individual to make a health decision. However:

- it is assumed that genuine freedom of choice exists; numerous people are not free to make a choice because of factors such as poverty, lack of education and low self-esteem
- the social, economic and political aspects of health are ignored
- the methods employed actually perpetuate inequalities, as often only the affluent have the time, money and education to make use of the health information given
- it is assumed that health professionals have the right to determine what is healthy behaviour; individual opinion and choice is ignored
- persuasive or coercive methods may be used to gain compliance
- total responsibility for health is placed on the individual; the individual is blamed for adopting an unhealthy

lifestyle when often the individual is not in a position to change

- as the professional sets the agenda, the individual is often not able to set his own goals

Doing good

The individual benefits from the professional passing on expert knowledge to which the individual will not normally have access. The individual then acts upon the information and adopts a healthy lifestyle, reducing his chances of becoming ill or dying early. However:

- few individuals are likely to change their behaviour in response to advice
- the arguments are often based on dubious evidence; for example, there is little evidence linking individual eating, drinking and exercising habits with the main forms of morbidity and mortality — the higher rates of coronary heart disease in the industrial world could be due to the long-term changes in the methods of food advertising, distribution and manufacture
- it is naive to assume that people automatically progress from gaining knowledge, to changing their attitude, to altering their behaviour; people usually make choices for more complex reasons

Doing no harm

It is assumed that no harm will come by persuading an individual to adopt a healthy lifestyle. However:

- the individual may feel guilty if he fails to follow advice
- false images and distorted values are often nurtured by misleading advertising campaigns

Being fair and equitable

Those with an 'unhealthy' lifestyle who are perceived to have the greater need are targeted. However:

- those individuals defined as high risk are often stigmatised

The ethos of the 'professional knows best' is also evident in the way health resources are sometimes rationed. For example, in many hospitals smokers are refused the option of heart bypass surgery because the rates of graft re-occlusion are significantly higher in smokers than in non-smokers. However, this is equating low mortality and morbidity rates with health. Even if the smoker only lives for 10 years after surgery, he may enjoy a greater sense of well-being than the non-smoker who lives for 15 years after surgery. It is possible that similar judgments could be made about other behaviours considered by health professionals to be risky or 'unhealthy'; for example asthmatics could be refused treatment if they smoke, or sports persons could be denied surgery to repair joint damage if they continue to play a high-impact sport.

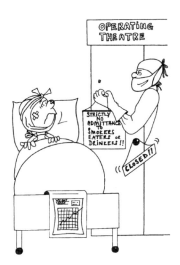

Educational approach

This approach is also based upon the belief that individuals should be held responsible for their health actions. Education is assumed to be a process whereby the individual learns about certain aspects of his health and then decides whether to alter his values and standards accordingly. The educator accepts the individual's health decision, irrespective of whether or not the educator agrees with the choice made. Knowledge is passed from the expert to the individual, and the agenda is again set by the expert.

This approach may be adopted, as on the surface it appears more ethically sound than the behaviour change model. For example, a midwife may decide to clarify the childbirth options open to a group of pregnant women, leaving the women then to come to their own decisions, rather than offering them her professional advice.

However, if the midwife's approach is adopted, how does this method abide by each of the ethical principles?

Respect for an individual's right to self-rule

The individual is allowed to make an informed choice and so his free will is protected. However:

- it is difficult to present information in a value-free way
- it is difficult for professionals not to express their own views
- it is assumed that genuine freedom of choice exists
- the social, economic and political dimensions of health are ignored
- inequalities are perpetuated as often only the affluent have the time, money and education to make use of the health information given
- total responsibility for health is placed on the individual

Doing good

The individual is benefited by the professional passing on expert knowledge to which the individual does not normally have access. However:

- the arguments are often based on dubious evidence

Doing no harm

Harm is prevented as the individual chooses whether or not to act on the information provided.

Being fair and equitable

Those with an 'unhealthy' lifestyle who are perceived to have the greater need are targeted. However:

- those individuals defined by professionals as high risk are often stigmatised

Therefore, unlike the behaviour change model, the educational model allows the individual to choose how to act on the health information provided. However, both models fail to address the issue that few individuals have genuine freedom of choice. With the example of the midwife, she may provide the same health information about childbirth to two pregnant mothers, but it may be that one lives in poverty in an inner city area and the other lives in comfort in an affluent area. The first mother may not have the education or social skills to apply this information in the same way that the second mother can.

Social change approach

There is a great deal of evidence to show that use of this approach can be beneficial for public health. Examples of successful programmes include legislation on family planning, compulsory wearing of seat belts and the fluoridation of public water supplies. *Health For All 2000* outlines the benefits of environmental, social and economic measures to reduce inequalities in health. Unlike the previous two approaches, this model recognises that deprivation is often the root of the problem. The health promoter takes on the role of the expert, protecting the people who are unable to help themselves.

It would appear that this approach has many benefits over the behaviour change and educational model. Structural barriers to health are both acknowledged and challenged. However, if nurses are involved in lobbying and campaigning for environmental and social change, are they still failing to comply with all of the ethical principles?

Respect for an individual's self-rule

The professional attempts to alter the social, environmental and political influences on health that are beyond the individual's control. However:

- the individual does not have freedom of choice because collective decisions are made
- by failing to involve the individual in the decision-making process, the professional prevents the individual from owning and feeling part of the action
- the professional may act 'paternally'; choosing to act on behalf of the individual for what is decided is for his benefit

Doing good

The healthy choice is made easier for individuals by the instigation of social, economic and political change. However:

- efforts are often hampered by influence of powerful lobbies, eg. agricultural and food industries
- legislative action often has a limited effect due to control of the larger vested interests of commerce and industry
- it is naive to place total responsibility for health on the state

Doing no harm

Harm is avoided as the structural barriers that prevent individuals from achieving health are minimised.

Being fair and equitable

The social injustices are addressed.

Thus, this approach tackles the structural barriers to health. A health visitor, campaigning locally for facilities for breast feeding in public places, is attempting to promote equal opportunities for women. However, the health visitor is acting paternalistically, addressing a need that exists according to her professional judgment. This need may not be recognised or attributed the same level of importance by the women in the local community. They may perceive their priority health needs to be the provision of practical local support in the form of free, drop-in, breast-feeding workshops.

Self-empowerment approach

This approach has developed relatively recently, within the last 15 years. The emphasis is on the individual's own defined health needs. The professional acts as a facilitator, enabling the individual to express and understand these health needs. The professional may also enable the individual to identify his own plan of health action. For example, many counselling services run on this basis.

The agenda is obviously set by the individual. There is also more of a partnership between the professional and the client in contrast to the hierarchical relationship adopted by the other approaches.

For example, a woman approaches a health visitor with some concerns about her weight. The health visitor may choose to use a self-empowerment approach and allow and encourage the client to discuss her concerns. By probing and facilitating the client to express her feelings, the health visitor enables the client to identify and understand her own eating habits. With help from the health visitor, the individual then sets a plan for some health actions.

Unlike the three previous approaches, this method empowers the individual and enables the client to retain self-control. However, this method still has its faults.

Respect for an individual's self-rule

Individuals are enabled to clarify their own health values and define their own health needs. However:

- the emphasis is still on the individual, and although it helps individuals to learn to cope with their circumstances, it does not address the social inequalities in health
- the individual may not wish to take responsibility for his health
- there is a danger that professionals focus on those individuals who are receptive and at ease with the notion of taking control. These are likely to be those in the higher social classes

In the main, though, the method is beneficial.

Doing good

The personal growth of the individual is facilitated.

Doing no harm

Harm is avoided by working from the individual's agenda.

Being fair and equitable

Individuals are equipped with the skills to deal with social injustices.

The self-empowerment approach allows the individual to retain autonomy and ownership of his health needs. It also enables the individual to develop his own coping strategies to deal with his health problems. The client mentioned previously, who is concerned about her weight, learns that she eats inappropriately primarily when she is stressed and unhappy. However, although the client can learn to develop other ways to cope with stress, the underlying problems — being out of work and short of money — are not directly addressed.

Community development approach

This approach shares many of the features of the self-empowerment model, except that it is on a larger scale. A group of individuals with similar health experiences work together to raise the profile of their concerns and to initiate change. The professional acts as a facilitator or as a resource. As a strategy for health promotion, this model is gaining popularity, especially within primary health care. It is also the main approach adopted in *Health For All 2000.* It appears to fit into the ethical framework more easily than the other approaches do.

Respect for an individual's self-rule

The group is enabled to clarify its common health values and define its shared health needs; resources are mobilised and the group is enabled to have a collective, potentially powerful voice. However:

- certain individuals may be allowed to dominate and dictate the agenda for the group
- instead of enabling the group to be proactive and to use their skills to negotiate positive health action, the group may be allowed to focus solely on the negative effects of the injustices of their position; this disables the group and fosters despondency

Doing good

Links are facilitated between individuals who share similar health needs; the personal growth of the individual is also facilitated.

Doing no harm

Harm is avoided by working from an agenda defined by the group.

Being fair and equitable

The power of the group voice is used to fight against social injustices.

For example, a nurse using the community development approach may facilitate a group of carers to work together to fight for their mental health needs. While this model does not directly set out to address the structural inequalities in health, part of this group's practice may involve campaigning and raising the profile of the needs of the underprivileged.

Going through the methods employed by each approach has highlighted some of the potential ethical dilemmas associated with the methods involved. Each approach has its place within the larger picture of health promotion practice. However, the type of approach must be chosen carefully, bearing in mind those actions that could have potentially harmful and self-limiting consequences for the clients involved.

Summary:

- there are four widely accepted ethical principles: respect for an individual's right to self-rule, doing good, doing no harm and being fair and equitable
- it is easy for nurses to abuse these principles because of the powerful position they assume as health professionals
- there are ethical dilemmas associated with each of the approaches to health education practice
- health professionals must work with patients and colleagues and choose the most appropriate method
- each approach has its place within the larger picture of health promotion practice

---

References

Beauchamp TL, Childress JF (1989) *Principles of Biomedical Ethics*. Oxford University Press, Oxford

Further reading

Ethics of health promotion

Allmark P (1995) Smoking and health: is discrimination fair? *Prof Nurse* **10**(12): 811–13
- This article discusses how decisions are made about the distribution of resources, and discusses the practice of refusing treatment to smokers

Beattie A (1991) Knowledge and control in health promotion: a test case for social policy and social theory. In: Gabe J, Calnan M, Bury M, eds. *The Sociology of The Health Service*. Routledge, London: 162–202
- This chapter explores conflicts in health promotion practice, using a structural map to examine each health promotion approach in turn

Caraher M (1995) Nursing and health education: victim blaming. *Br J Nurs* **4**(20): 1190–213
- This article explores the concept of victim blaming and outlines concerns with the adoption of a behaviour change approach

Clarke J (1993) Ethical issues in health education. *Br J Nurs* **2**(10): 533–8
- The article examines the four ethical principles and relates them to nurse decision making. The example of screening is used to highlight dilemmas in practice

Cribb A (1993) Health promotion — a human science. In: Wilson-Barnett J, Macleod Clark J, eds. *Research in Health Promotion and Nursing*. Macmillan Press, Hampshire: 29–35
- The author raises ethical concerns about health promotion being used as a mechanism of social control

Cribb A, Dines A (1993) Ethical issues in health promotion. In: Dines A, Cribb A, eds. *Health Promotion: Concepts and Practice*. Blackwell Science Ltd, Oxford:46–64
- This chapter provides practical examples of ethical dilemmas in health promotion practice

DeBreu D (1995) Implications of smoking bans in long-term care. *Prof Nurse* **11**(1): 44–5
● This article questions whether smoking bans deny patients of their rights to make their own choices

Dines A (1993) A case study of ethical issues in health promotion — mammography screening: the nurse's position. In: Wilson-Barnett J, Macleod Clark J, eds. *Research in Health Promotion and Nursing*. Macmillan Press, Hampshire: 43–50
● This chapter explores the ethical issues faced by a nurse who adopts different approaches to health education, using mammography as an example

Downie RS, Fyfe C, Tannahill A (1990) *Health Promotion: Models and Values*. Oxford Medical Publications, Oxford
● This book provides a theoretical insight into the philosophical aspects of health promotion

Ewles L, Simnett I (1992) *Promoting Health: A Practical Guide*, 2nd edn. Scutari, London
● Chapter three explores philosophical issues inherent in health promotion practice in simple terms

Farrant W, Russell J (1986) *The Politics of Health Information: Beating Heart Disease as a Case Study of Health Education Council Publications*. Bedford Way Papers 28, Institute of Education, University of London, London
● The authors argue for increased recognition of the importance of social and economic factors in coronary heart disease

Jacob F (1994) Ethics in health promotion: freedom or determinism. *Br J Nurs* **3**(6): 299–302
● This article explores nurses' beliefs about human nature and the influence that these beliefs have on their approach to the promotion of health

Lask S (1992a) Health promotion: a question of choice. *Nurs Times* **88**(7 Open Learning Programme): i–viii
● This article discusses different approaches to health promotion and questions how much control people have over their health

Lask S (1992b) Issues and dilemmas. *Nurs Times* **88**(8;7 Open Learning Programme): ii–vii
● This article discusses different approaches to health education in nursing practice and the common problems encountered

Naidoo J, Wills J (1994) *Health Promotion: Foundations for Practice*. Bailliere Tindall, London
- Chapter six discusses ethical decision-making in health promotion practice

Rodmell S, Watt A, eds (1986) *The Politics of Health Education: Raising the Issues*. Routledge and Kegan Paul, London
- This book provides a critical analysis of individualistic approaches to health education

Seedhouse D (1988) *Ethics: The Heart of Health Care*. John Wiley and Sons Ltd, London
- This book explores the philosophy of health and provides a detailed theoretical basis for understanding how ethics and health care are interlinked

Whitehead M (1989) *Swimming Upstream. Trends and Prospects in Education for Health*. King's Fund, London
- This document questions the effectiveness of mass media campaigns and discusses major obstacles to health education by nurses

Chapter 4

Health promotion in nursing

Having examined the contextual aspects of health promotion, consideration will now be given to its relationship with nursing.

This chapter covers:

- Research in health promotion and nursing
- The importance of health promotion in nursing
- The role of the nurse in health education
- The position of the nurse as a role model for health
- The nurse–patient relationship: health education on a micro level

Research in health promotion and nursing

The number of articles and research focusing on health promotion and nursing is on the increase. There is still scope for further research focusing on the use of health promotion in nursing practice.

Most recent research articles concentrate on an examination of one of the following aspects:

- *outcome measures*; the extent or impact of various health promotion initiatives on individuals' behaviour or attitudes
- factors that *influence* health promotion practice
- nurses' *abilities* to act as health educators
- patients' *perceptions* of health promotion practice
- nurses' *attitudes and beliefs* about the concept and practice of health promotion

At the outset it is important to establish what operational definition of health promotion is being used in any particular study. Frequently the author concerned has restricted the focus to 'health education' alone, whereas health education and health promotion are different concepts and the terms should not be used interchangeably. Again, the different strategies of both need to be borne in mind; for example, the term health education may be taken to equate solely with an individualistic, behaviour change type of approach, whereas strategies which promote health may be linked with a social change or community development approach.

The importance of health promotion in nursing

The drive to incorporate health promotion into nursing practice is currently assuming a high profile in the nursing press. This could be regarded as a passing fad. Alternatively, it could be seen as an acknowledgement that promoting the health of an individual is an essential aspect of caring, requiring skills, which if mastered, contribute greatly to the art of nursing.

Widespread recognition of the importance of the role of the nurse in health promotion practice has originated from various quarters: notably the Department of Health, the United Kingdom Central Council for Nursing, Midwifery and

Health Visiting (UKCC), and the English National Board (ENB).

The main initiatives acknowledging the role of health promotion in nursing:

Professionally driven

- *health promotion is top of the list of competencies for the first-level nurse.* In 1983, following the *Nurses, Midwives and Health Visitors Act* (Department of Health, 1979), the registered nurse training changed. Rule 18 stipulates that, in order to qualify for admission to the register, the student nurse must acquire several competencies, the first of which is the competency required to 'advise on the promotion of health and the prevention of illness'

- *The UKCC's Code of Professional Conduct (UKCC, 1992) draws attention to the role of the nurse as the client's advocate.* Clauses one and five detail that, as part of her professional accountability for her practice, the nurse must promote the interests of clients and work with clients fostering their involvement in their care

- *A Vision for the Future* (Department of Health, 1993a) states that members of the nursing professions have the ability not only to empower individuals, but also to influence the environments in which individuals live and work

Educationally driven

- *Project 2000, diploma and degree courses have incorporated health promotion into their curricula*

Politically driven

- *The Patient's Charter* (Department of Health, 1991) has prompted clients to expect to be involved in their own care and take more responsibility for their health.

- The '*Health of the Nation*' (Department of Health, 1992) identifies hospitals, schools, homes, industry and other community groupings as important in the process of improving the health of the population

In addition, there has been a general process of consciousness-raising within the nursing profession itself. Attention has focused on defining the intricacies of the nurse's role. The roles of the specialist practitioner and the advanced practitioner are developing to incorporate the exploration of nursing boundaries, the advancement of practice and the strengthening of client control in their own care.

The exact role of the nurse as health promoter has received similar debate. The nursing literature acknowledges the limitations of the behaviour change and educational models for health education practice. It is not surprising then to note that educationalists are calling for nurses to inform and enable clients to take control of their own health. In response to *Health For All 2000*, educationalists have also focused on the role of the nurse as the patient's advocate and called for nurses to fight for equality for all.

Summary:

- the UKCC, ENB and the Department of Health have all acknowledged the importance of the nurse's role in health promotion practice
- within the nursing profession there has been much discussion on the exact nature of the nurse's role in health education/promotion practice
- educationalists have called for nurses to empower clients and to fight for equality for all

The role of the nurse in health education

Empowerment in practice: the successes

The benefits of holistic and client-centered care are recognised in nursing theory. Over the last 10 years there have been a number of changes in the working practices of nurses, health visitors and midwives that have actively encouraged client participation in care. Initiatives such as *The Named Nurse, Midwife and Health Visitor* (Department of Health, 1993b) and *Changing Childbirth* (Department of Health, 1993c) have been introduced to increase client contact with a named professional. Primary nursing also works on the basis of a participatory partnership between the nurse and the patient.

Some health professionals working with clients on a one-to-one basis will also find themselves enabling the individual to take control. For example, the terminally ill client may feel overwhelmed by a sense of powerlessness. The Macmillan nurse can play an enormously beneficial role by initially providing the client with information about his health, thus allowing the client to feel some measure of control even if this is only to anticipate future events. The nurse can also allow and assist the client to identify the issues that are causing him concern. After the individual has identified what support he requires, the nurse can then mobilise the appropriate resources; for instance, the nurse can put the client in touch with a self-help group and arrange for him to have a complementary therapy such as massage.

Many community-based nurses are already involved in the process of empowering individuals and groups. For example, the school nurse may respond to teenagers' requests and set up a workshop entitled 'Resisting the urge to smoke' aimed at exploring ways for them to withstand pressure from their peers. A health visitor may facilitate a self-help group for mothers with postnatal depression.

The importance of working with groups in the community to define local needs is also being recognised. This may mean involving community groups in the process and evaluation of patient literature or patient information projects. It may also include establishing client focus groups to enable patients and their families to identify their particular priorities for meeting local health needs. Feedback from the community about the nature and quality of service provision may also be beneficial.

Empowerment in practice: the difficulties

However, there can be a number of difficulties associated with trying to incorporate a self-empowerment or community development approach into nursing practice:

- there is little preparation for the knowledge and skills necessary to undertake this role both in the traditional form of nurse education and in current pre-registration courses. The result is that:
  - ✛ the majority of nurses have not had the opportunity to examine their own values and beliefs about their role as health promoters; a team of nurses may not have discussed and chosen a shared philosophy for their health education practice. This means that the service they provide is likely to be fragmented and confusing for the client
  - ✛ few nurses are sufficiently self-aware and confident to facilitate the self-discovery of others
- due to other priorities, some nurses do not have the time available to spend working closely with one client; others may not work in a suitable environment
- the client himself may not actually wish to be put in a situation where he can take control of his health

The following examples illustrate this:
- a team of health visitors take it in turn to run a healthy eating clinic. One health visitor makes it clear that her role is not to provide medical advice, but to allow clients to explore their eating patterns and to provide the necessary support they require. However, the following week another health visitor then lightly scolds those clients who have not adhered to a medically defined dietary plan.
- a district nurse has been involved with an elderly woman's care over a length of time. The nurse has built up a close relationship with the client and gradually allows the client to explore some of her feelings. The client starts to express emotions such as anger and acute distress. The nurse then feels uncomfortable and threatened by the client's behaviour. She is unsure how to respond on a professional and personal level.

- a coronary care nurse has been working with a group of clients and their spouses who have come together to share their experiences and provide support for one another. The mood within the group becomes very negative and self-destructive. One member becomes abusive and critical of the care he received in hospital. The nurse feels unsure how to handle this situation and becomes anxious and defensive
- a nurse working on a busy medical ward has built up a rapport with one of her patients who is recovering from a heart attack. She also has eight other patients to care for during shift. She is likely to prioritise the relief of pain and the administration of pressure relief for her other patients above the practise of health education for this patient
- a midwife works with a mother to enable the woman to take control of her health. The midwife explains the choices available, but the mother is unhappy about making a decision; she would rather be advised by a health professional who she thinks knows what is best for her

In addition, in order to enable the process where a client moves from a position where the professional makes most of his health decisions to a position where the client starts taking control of his own health, the culture and working environment must actively encourage and support the taking of this risk. However, nurses, midwives and health visitors do not work in isolation; they frequently work as part of the larger, multidisciplinary team. Other members of the team may not share the same values and beliefs and may be working towards different outcomes of health education practice.

For example, a rehabilitation nurse may spend some time with a woman while she discusses her anxieties about her smoking habits. The patient may assess her life and decide that despite the harmful effects of the habit, what is healthy for her is to carry on smoking as it gives her pleasure and provides a means of relaxation. By providing the patient with an opportunity to talk through her fears the nurse has enabled the woman to achieve a positive health outcome.

However, the GP may see this interaction as a negative outcome as the woman still intends to smoke.

This problem is accentuated within the hospital setting. The culture of an organisation is largely determined by the values and beliefs of those in senior positions. Thus, the belief and value that those in powerful positions, such as hospital managers and doctors, attach to the role of the nurse as an autonomous practitioner must be demonstrable in practice. If the nurse is not empowered herself, then she is not going to be in a position to empower others. While it is acknowledged that midwives and nurses working in primary health care are less constrained by these managerial and medical power relations, it is likely that GPs or practice managers may still have a strong influence over service provision.

Social change in practice: the difficulties

It has been acknowledged that certain social and economic structures disable and prevent certain individuals and groups from achieving their health goals. Social change usually comes about as a result of the following:

- the creation of healthy public policies
- lobbying
- the setting of agendas based on local health needs
- awareness raising campaigns

Health professionals can also help by adopting the role of:

- mediator between groups with different interests
- advocate for disadvantaged groups

Nurses traditionally have not been used to adopting these roles. Their education and training does not prepare them for a social change approach. In addition, political activity within the nursing profession has been frowned upon.

While it is unlikely that many nurses will base their health education practice solely on the social change model, they need to be encouraged to consider the wider, structural influences on health.

Setting new targets

In chapter three, the importance of recognising that health education can use a wide variety of complementary strategies was discussed. All the health education strategies should be recognised as having their own degree of importance. When nurses use a particular approach they need to bear in mind the ethical implications of their actions.

Although the drawbacks of a behaviour change approach need to be acknowledged, nurses should be careful not to set their sights in health education practice too high. They must be very careful not to label their practice as self-empowerment when in reality they are using their professional position of power to influence the client. Likewise, the term 'participation' must not be confused with empowerment. A client may participate in his care, but, without the necessary skills and resources to influence his health, he is in a relatively powerless position.

At its simplest level, the aim of health education practice for nurses should be to:

- Strive for an 'unconditional acceptance' of the individual's health values
- Show consideration of the environmental and social factors affecting the individual
- Offer health information, though not in the form of indoctrination, advice or persuasion. Nurses need to be aware that it is almost impossible to give information which is totally void of a value judgment. Therefore, they must develop their communication skills and examine their position as providers of information. Because they are perceived as credible and authoritative by the public, they have a responsibility to provide up-to-date, accurate health information

Health education practice aimed at the individual should take the form of:

- valuing the individual and the individual's health beliefs
- showing sensitivity to the environmental, social and economic factors affecting the health status of the individual
- providing health information
- constantly evaluating and reviewing the accuracy of available health information
- raising the individual's awareness of the social, economic and environmental determinants of health
- informing the individual of his rights
- involving the individual in decision making where possible
- offering support to the individual and mobilising appropriate resources; making contacts and links with appropriate professionals
- respecting the individual's right to choose his course of health action
- uniting with other nurses to ensure that professional bodies lobby for healthy public policy

These themes also need to be reflected in a strategy for health education practice for community development.

Health education practice for community development should take the form of:

- establishing and valuing the predominant health beliefs that exist within the local community
- showing sensitivity to the local environmental, social and economic factors affecting the health status of the community
- providing health information
- constantly evaluating and reviewing the accuracy of available health information
- raising the community's awareness of the social, economic and environmental determinants of health
- informing the community of their rights

- establishing local health needs and the community's priorities for action
- involving the community in decision making and the provision of health action
- offering professional support for community groups, mobilising appropriate resources, providing inter-agency links
- uniting with other nurses and community groups to lobby for healthy public policy

Summary:

- some nurses are in a position to empower clients either on an individual basis or on a community development basis
- other nurses may find it difficult to use these health education strategies as they may not have the skills or self-confidence required, they may not feel in a position of power themselves, and their work environment may actually militate against clients taking control
- nurses in general find it difficult to incorporate a social change approach into their nursing practice
- nurses should not set their sights in health education practice too high
- provided it is used with consideration, each approach has its place within nursing practice

The position of the nurse as a role model for health

In their role as health professionals, most nurses at one time or other have come under pressure to act as role models for health behaviour. This pressure originates from the belief that nurses are only credible if they display signs of self-discipline and demonstrate a commitment to positive health actions. In other words, a nurse will lose a client's trust if she displays signs of negative health actions, ie. smells of smoke, appears unkempt or is overweight.

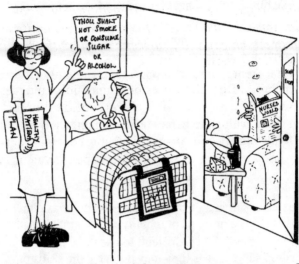

However, is it realistic or right to expect nurses to adopt the position of role model for health, both professionally and personally? Should all nurses be non-smokers, exercise regularly, eat a low fat, low sugar, high fibre diet, practise safe sex and manage stress effectively?

These expectations are both unrealistic and misplaced because:

- these positive and negative health outcomes are medically defined; the nurse may feel healthy despite the fact that she smokes
- the philosophy underlying this expectation assumes that health is wholly within the control of the individual and that nurses have the freedom of choice to change their behaviour if they so desire

'[My colleagues] insisted that I had a duty to be a healthy role model...and to be one you must not drink alcohol and coffee or smoke cigarettes (or anything else for that matter), or eat much red meat or sausage or bacon or too much of anything else. One should work but not too much or too little. One should marry (neither too young nor too old), have children (neither too many nor too few), go to bed and arise about the same time each day,

exercise regularly, remain geographically stable, and avoid noise, crowds and white bread and white sugar (both of which cause a gruesome death within hours of ingestion)' (Curtin, 1986).

A nurse's credibility should be demonstrable in practice. If a nurse is at ease with herself; if she is confident and skilled at interpersonal relationships; if she inspires trust with her speech and body language; and if she communicates with warmth and empathy, then she will be perceived as credible.

Summary:

* nurses are often expected to act as role models for health behaviour
* this health behaviour is medically defined
* nurses' credibility originates from their practice

The nurse–patient relationship: health education on a micro level

In the first chapter, it is acknowledged that health has a relevance for everyone. Thus, the potential for health promotion can be perceived on a vast scale. On the macro level, promoting health for both individuals and communities can encompass such activities as legislation and campaigning for health, implementation of further welfare benefits, disclosure of health information, and social skills training. However, on a micro level, something as small as an interaction between two people can be seen to affect the health of either person.

How many times each day are people in a position to affect the well-being of another individual? Numerous times, either directly, eg. affording time to listen to a friend talk through a problem, or indirectly, eg. disposing of a glass bottle correctly, rather than leaving it in a public place where a child could injure himself. Nurses not only play a part in promoting health within their professional lives, they also promote the health of others, primarily those they care about, every day in their personal lives.

This theme is touched upon in the first chapter, where it is noted that health promotion can be perceived as a set of particular values. These values then underpin how an individual thinks, speaks and behaves. In order to strive for health for all, importance must be afforded to the following:

- holism — considering the patient as a whole, taking into account the inter-related and inter-dependant aspects of his person
- equality — ensuring the standard of care is the same for each patient, despite obvious differences in gender, age, class, creed, race, etc
- autonomy — respecting and adhering to the patient's choices where possible

These humanistic values also underpin the practice of *caring*. In other words, some of the key building blocks which enable nurses to promote health are also considered central to nursing. The caring relationship between nurse and patient therefore has great potential for promoting the well-being of the patient (and to some extent, the nurse).

However, each nurse will carry her own *world view* about the nature of health and health promotion. It is not possible to legislate for the management of each nurse–patient interaction. Nurses are in a powerful position as health professionals and as such have the potential to stifle patients' capacity for personal growth or adversely affect their sense of well-being. The most obvious example would be if the nurse abused her position of power to influence the patient's health choices.

The value of autonomy is of great importance for the promotion of health. To be autonomous, an individual needs to be able to:

- understand his environment and circumstances

- make rational choices
- act on these choices

It is evident from previous discussions that few individuals are in a position of autonomy due to external conditions over which they have little control. In hospital, this problem is intensified, because of the structure and operation of the organisation. However, the nurse can influence the level of bureaucracy and has some control over the nature of her interaction with the patient. Establishing a relationship based on trust, partnership, mutual respect and collaboration shifts the power base from the professional to the patient.

For example, a ward may practise primary nursing. This system of care offers continuity of care to the patient and encourages the nurse to take responsibility for the patient throughout the patient's stay in hospital. If the ward staff share a philosophy of equality, participation and partnership, then this is likely to be evident in the primary nurse's practice. If the primary nurse receives the support and guidance required from the ward manager, then she may feel empowered herself to allow the patient to take control over aspects of care.

Schemes such as self-medication in hospital enable patients to take responsibility for their drugs while in hospital. The patients are provided with detailed information about their drugs. They are also given the support they require from the nurses and pharmacists. The patients therefore take control over the administration of their medication which may allow them to feel some vestige of control over their health.

Obviously clients who acquire certain competences can exert influence over the pattern of events. For example, a mother may learn relaxation skills to help reduce her labour pains.

Even the simple nurse–patient interaction is important. Interaction with patients can be of the verbal or non-verbal form. Non-verbal communication is of great importance. For example, in a certain situation the use of direct eye contact, touch and nodding of the head may indicate the health professional's interest and warmth, which in turn may encourage the patient to feel valued and able to express his own opinions. Similarly, avoidance of eye contact or disapproval on the face of the health professional may prevent the patient from feeling able to voice his thoughts.

Examples of verbal communication		
providing information	humouring	empathising
reinforcing information	clarifying	exploring
discussing	reflecting	supporting
acknowledging	questionning	

Examples of non-verbal communication
facial expression, such as direct eye contact, smiling, nodding
active listening
body language, such as touching

With any interaction, it is virtually impossible for health professionals to avoid imposing their own health values onto the patient. When a midwife engages in light conversation about her interest in music to the mother, these values are regarded as an important indicator of the midwife's self, and provide insight into her personal life.

However, when health information is passed from the professional to the patient, the effect of these values may be more significant. If the facts are clear-cut and understood by the health professional, the exchange of information may occur with little problem, for example the midwife will probably find it easy to pass on information about the cardioprotective benefits of breast feeding for the baby. If the information is, however, vague and conflicting, for example the relationship between mammography and the detection of breast cancer, the nurse may be more likely to introduce her own beliefs about the subject.

Interaction is often not only restricted to the giving of health information, but also encompasses the giving of advice. Due to the knowledge the health professional holds, she is in a position of relative power in relation to the client. A professional is often in a position of influence because she is perceived as credible and trustworthy by the public.

But there are obvious concerns about this role of giving advice:

- with the case of the nurse informing the patient about the role of mammography, there is little statistical evidence to suggest that breast cancer screening reduces mortality rates. The nurse, however, may herself believe that screening is beneficial, and this judgment may be evident in her delivery of the information. The patient may be left with an unbalanced picture of the situation
- with the case of the midwife, as well as being aware of the facts, she may feel very strongly about the benefits of breast feeding. In this case, she may stop giving information and start persuading the mother to choose to breast feed
- in any situation where the health professional works from her own agenda, the social situation, culture and personality make-up of the patient is ignored

It is easy to see that different types of interaction can take place which actually disempower the individual, including:

- persuading
- scolding
- expressing approval
- expressing disapproval
- directing

However, it is also not sufficient for health professionals merely to pass on information. Health professionals also have a responsibility to place this information within the context of the individual's cultural setting, and to consider the individual's beliefs, attitudes and values. Each person's health behaviour is different to the next.

People also adopt lifestyles for personal reasons and attach value to their behaviour. Most individuals can identify a friend or member of their family who lived to a great age yet smoked and drank excessive amounts. Others will be able to identify a colleague who exercised regularly and gave up eating meat, yet was miserable and unhealthy in their eyes.

There are certain theories that have been suggested to explain lay health behaviours.

Theories of health behaviour:

- The *Health Belief Model* (Becker, 1974) suggests that an individual will only take health actions if certain conditions are present:
  - ✛ certain cues must be present to create a situation in which an individual may consider taking a health action, eg. a pregnancy may provoke a woman into considering giving up smoking
  - ✛ whether this action is then taken up depends on the person's perception of the threats and benefits involved, eg. the pleasures of smoking for the mother *vs* the risk she perceives to the unborn baby

- The *Locus of Control* (Wallston and Wallston, 1978) theory suggests that individuals differ in their beliefs as to how much of their health is actually due to fate. If an individual believes that his pattern of health is predetermined, then he is less likely to want to take control

- The *Attribution Theory* (Abramson *et al*, 1978). This suggests that during an illness, people may try to gain control over the situation by attempting to understand why the illness or event occurred and what impact it will have. The individual's perceptions about the cause of the event may determine how the individual responds and feels

Summary:

- the relationship between the health professional and patient is an important tool in the promotion of health for the patient. Depending on the character of the interaction, the professional can maximise the patient's perception of control
- it is important for nurses to be aware of their values and beliefs and how these can affect the delivery of information to a client
- clients have their own values which affect their health behaviour; in order for nurses to work effectively with clients, they must try to gain an understanding of these lay beliefs

References

Abramson LY, Seligman MEP, Teasdale JD (1978) Learned helplessness in humans: critique and reformulation. *J Abnormal Psychol* **87**: 49–74

Becker MH (1974) The health belief model and personal health behaviour. *Health Educ Monographs* **2**: 324–508

Curtin LL (1986) The case of the reluctant role model: from health to heresy. *Nurs Man* **17**(7): 7–8

Department of Health (1979) *Nurses, Midwives and Health Visitors Act*. HMSO, London

Department of Health (1991) *The Patient's Charter*. HMSO, London

Department of Health (1992) *The Health of Nation: A Strategy for Health in England*. HMSO, London

Department of Health (1993a) *A Vision for the Future: The Nursing, Midwifery and Health Visiting Contribution to Health and Healthcare*. NHS Management Executive, London

Department of Health (1993b) *The Named Nurse, Midwife and Health Visitor*. NHS Management Executive, London

Department of Health (1993c) *Changing Childbirth*. Report of the Expert Maternity Group, HMSO, London

English National Board (1985) *Professional education/training courses*. Consultation Paper. ENB , London

United Kingdom Central Council for Nursing, Midwifery and Health Visiting (1986) *Project 2000: A New Preparation for Practice*. UKCC, London

United Kingdom Central Council for Nursing, Midwifery and Health Visiting (1992) *Code of Professional Conduct for the Nurse, Midwife and Health Visitor*. UKCC, London

Wallston KA, Wallston BS (1978) Health locus of control. *Health Educ Monographs* **6**: 2

Further reading

Research in health promotion and nursing

Gott M, O'Brien M (1990a) Attitudes and beliefs in health promotion. *Nurs Standard* **5**(2): 30–2
- This study used interviews and non-participant observation of nurses (including health visitors, district nurses and practice nurses) to gain an understanding of their perceptions and practices of health promotion

Johnston I (1988) *A Study of the Promotion of Healthy Lifestyles by Hospital-Based Staff*. Unpublished MSc thesis, University of Birmingham
- The author interviewed patients on general surgical wards to obtain their perceptions of the health education they had received. Nursing documentation was also examined

Latter S, Macleod-Clark J, Wilson-Barnett J, Maben J (1992) Health education in nursing: perceptions of practice in acute settings. *J Adv Nurs* **17**: 164–72
- This study used a postal survey to establish senior nurses perceptions of health education practice in general ward settings

Mackintosh N (1993) *Nurses and their Role in Health Promotion: Inconsistencies between Theory and Practice?* Unpublished MSc thesis, University of Central England in Birmingham
- The author used a postal survey to examine hospital-based nurses' perceptions of the concept and role of health education and health promotion

Macleod-Clark J, Haverty S, Kendall S (1990) Helping people to give up smoking: a study of the nurse's role. *J Adv Nurs* **15**: 357–63

- This study used a case-study approach to describe the process and assess the outcome of nurses' attempts to help clients stop smoking

Tilley JD, Gregor FM, Thiessen V (1987) The nurse's role in patient education: incongruent perceptions among nurses and patients. *J Adv Nurs* **12**: 291–301

- This study used a nurse questionnaire and a patient interview schedule to ascertain similarities and differences in perceptions between nurses and patients of the nurse's role in health education

Wilson-Barnett J, Macleod Clark J, eds (1993) *Research in Health Promotion and Nursing*. Macmillan Press, Hampshire

- This book includes details of several important research studies

The role of the nurse in health education

Campbell AV (1993) The ethics of health education. In: Wilson-Barnett J, Macleod Clark J eds. *Research in Health Promotion and Nursing*. Macmillan Press, Hampshire: 20–8

- The author challenges nursing as a profession to break with its traditional individualistic approach. Instead he urges it to confront the social injustices of health

Denny E, Jacob F (1990) Defining health promotion. Senior Nurse 10(10): 7–9

- The authors question the future of health visiting if it persists with its focus on the needs of the individual and argue for a collective, collaborative approach to health promotion in the community

Gallagher U, Burden J (1993) Nursing as health promotion — a myth accepted? In: Wilson-Barnett J, Macleod Clark J, eds. *Research in Health Promotion and Nursing*. The Macmillan Press, Hampshire: 51–8

- The authors argue that the values and beliefs that underpin nursing are in conflict with the philosophical framework of health promotion

Gott M, O'Brien M (1990b) The role of the nurse in health promotion. *Health Promot Intl* **5**(2): 137–43

- This article discusses the legitimacy and development of a health promotion role in nursing

Keyzer DM (1988) Challenging role boundaries: conceptual frameworks for understanding the conflict arising from the implementation of the nursing process in practice. In: White R, ed. *Political Issues in Nursing: Past, Present and Future*, Vol 3. John Wiley and Sons, Chichester: 95–119
- The author discusses the traditional occupational strategy that is predominant in nursing which refers decision making upwards

Mackintosh N (1995) Self-empowerment in health promotion: a realistic target? *Br J Nurs* **4**(21): 1273–8
- This article details the difficulties associated with implementation of a self-empowerment approach in nursing

Macleod Clark J (1993) From sick nursing to health nursing: evolution or revolution? In: Wilson-Barnett J, Macleod Clark J, eds. *Research in Health Promotion and Nursing*. Macmillan Press, Hampshire: 256–70
- This chapter explores the different philosophy to care embodied in sick nursing and health nursing and advocates a move towards the latter

Mitchell L (1989) Whose health for all? *Nurs Times* **85**(34): 48–50
- A thought-provoking challenge as to whether *Health For All* assumes an unrealistic political position. The article questions the motive behind nursing's enthusiasm to embrace a health promotion focus

Myer J (1993) Lay participation in care: threat to the status quo. In: Wilson-Barnett J, Macleod Clark J, eds. *Research in Health Promotion and Nursing*. Macmillan Press, Hampshire: 86–100
- This chapter details the conflict and problems encountered with a project designed to increase lay participation in care

Naish J (1995) Ethics and accountability in health visiting. *Br J Nurs* **4**(11): 659–63
- This article argues for health visitors to adopt a community development approach to maintain a standard for ethical practice

Roberts SJ, Krouse HJ (1990) Negotiation as a strategy to empower self-care. *Holistic Nurs Pract* **4**(2): 30–6
- This article explores self-care as a method of empowerment and discusses difficulties with the implementation of self-care in health-care settings

Robinson J (1985) Health visiting and health. In: White R, ed. *Political Issues in Nursing: Past, Present and Future.* John Wiley and Sons, Chichester: 67–86

- This chapter explores the notion that although health visitors are encouraged to operate from the ideal of collective health they operate their collective theories only at the level of the individual

Salvage J (1992) The new nursing: empowering patients or empowering nurses? In: Robinson J, Gray A, Elkin R, eds. *Policy Issues in Nursing.* Open University Press, Milton Keynes: 9–23

- This chapter presents a critical analysis of the role of the new practitioner in nursing and explores the social and organisational constraints to the implementation of patient-centered care

Tones BK (1990) The power to choose — health education and the new public health. *J Inst Health Educ* **28**(3): 73–9

- The author provides support of the individualistic role in health education

Williams S (1990) Motivating self-care: A nursing approach. *Holistic Nurs Pract* **4**(12): 13–21

- This article discusses theories of motivation and health behaviour and details how nurses can use theory to promote self-care in practice

The position of the nurse as a role model for health

Clarke AC (1991) Nurses as role models and health educators. *J Adv Nurs* **16**: 1178–84

- This article provides a comprehensive review of the concept of the nurse as a role model for health and the expectations placed on nurses from within and outside the profession

Melvin B (1987) Promoting health by example. *Nurs Times* **83**: 42–3

- This author argues for the nurse to act as a role model for health

Noble C (1991) Are nurses good patient educators? *J Adv Nurs* **16**: 1185–9

- This article discusses the nurse's role as patient educator and highlights concerns that nurses often lack the skills, knowledge, motivation and support required for this role

Theories of health behaviour

Bennett P, Hodgson R (1992) Psychology and health promotion:
In: Bunton R, Macdonald G, eds. *Health Promotion:
Disciplines and Diversity*. Routledge, London and New York:
23–41
- This chapter explores the psychological theories which have
provided explanations for health behaviour

Davison C (1994) Conflicts of interest. *Nurs Times* **90**(13): 40–2
- This article discusses some of the social and cultural reasons why
people behave in certain ways

Naidoo J, Wills J (1994) *Health Promotion: Foundations for
Practice*. Bailliere Tindall, London
- Chapter ten looks at theoretical models used to explain changes in
behaviour

Chapter 5

Health of the Nation

Although the *Health of the Nation* (Department of Health, 1992) as a working strategy for health has already been mentioned in chapter two, this book would not be complete without a more detailed examination of its practical application. The strategy identifies a clear role for nurses, midwives and health visitors to help achieve its objectives and targets. Indeed, the document *Targeting Practice: the Contribution of Nurses, Midwives and Health Visitors* (Department of Health, 1993) has already noted examples of good practice to date where various nurses have participated in projects designed to help meet the targets outlined.

This chapter addresses the following:
- The key areas
- The targets for action
- A philosophy of *Health of the Nation*
- The strategy as a behaviour change approach
- The strategy in the form of a self-empowerment approach
- The strategy in the form of a social change approach
- The strategy in the form of a community development approach

The key areas

The idea behind the White Paper as a public strategy for health should to be welcomed. It focuses attention on the nation's health, and publicly demonstrates commitment towards the promotion of health in society.

The *Health of the Nation* focuses on five key areas where the need for improvements is perceived as greatest, and where long-lasting success is considered to be most likely to be achieved. The five key areas are:

- coronary heart disease and stroke
- cancers
- mental illness
- immunodeficiency virus (HIV)/acquired immunodeficiency (AIDS) and sexual health
- accidents

Each key area:

- is a major cause of serious illness or early death; it could be regarded as an area of the greatest need
- offers scope for effective action
- offers scope for targets that can be set and measured

The targets for action

The Government's strategy identifies targets for action for each of the key areas.

Targets for coronary heart disease and stroke
(Department of Health, 1992)

By the year 2000 to:

- reduce heart disease death rates in people under 65 years by at least 40%, and among people between 65 and 74 years by at least 30%

- reduce the death rate from stroke among people under 75 years by at least 40%
- reduce the number of people smoking by about a third

By the year 2005 to:

- reduce the number of people aged 16 to 64 years who are obese by at least a quarter for men and at least a third for women
- reduce average intake of fat by 12% and saturates by 35%
- reduce the number of men drinking more than 21 units of alcohol per week and women drinking more than 14 units per week by a third
- reduce mean systolic blood pressure in the adult population by at least 5 mm Hg

Some of the targets are based on the reduction of mortality rates and some focus on specific behaviours.

Targets for cancers (Department of Health, 1992)

By the year 2000 to:

- reduce the number of people smoking by about a third
- reduce the rate of breast cancer deaths among women invited for screening by at least 25%
- reduce the incidence of invasive cervical cancer by approximately 20%

By the year 2005 to:

- halt the increase in the incidence of skin cancer

By the year 2010 to:

- reduce the rate of lung cancer deaths by at least 30% in men and by at least 15% in women under the age of 75 years

'Mental illness' covers conditions such as schizophrenia, affective psychosis, depression, anxiety states and dementia.

Targets for mental illness (Department of Health, 1992)

- to improve significantly the health and social functioning of mentally ill people

By the year 2000 to:

- reduce the overall suicide rate by at least 15%
- reduce the suicide rate of severely mentally ill people by at least 33%

Specific targets for HIV and AIDS have not been set as the time delay between transmission of the disease and the onset of symptoms or diagnosis has made it difficult to establish a baseline figure from which to work. Thus the number of unwanted pregnancies, the amount of drug misuse and the amount of people suffering from sexually transmitted diseases has been targeted.

Targets for sexual health (Department of Health, 1992)

By the year 2000 to:

- reduce the rate of conceptions among those under 16 years by at least 50%
- reduce the percentage of injected drug misusers who report sharing injecting equipment in the previous 4 weeks by at least 50% by 1997, and by at least a further 50% by the year 2000

The scope for accident prevention covers a variety of age groups.

Targets for Accidents (Department of Health, 1992)

By the year 2005 to:

- reduce the death rate for accidents among children aged under 15 years by at least 33%
- reduce the death rate for accidents among young people aged 15–24 years by at least 25%

- reduce the death rate for accidents among people aged 65 years and over by at least 33%

A philosophy of *Health of the Nation*

From these key areas and targets for action it is evident that:

- while *Health of the Nation* outwardly states that its purpose is to enhance health, it is actually only working towards reducing ill-health
- the needs and targets are based on epidemiological data, ie. reducing death rates or incidence rates
- the *Health of the Nation* incorporates the biomedical view of health
- there are other priority groups with particular health needs which have escaped attention, such as the elderly or those with a drug or alcohol addiction

Thus it can be seen that *Health of the Nation* is a strategy based on the behaviour change model. Its success is largely dependent on the achievement of individual lifestyle change.

The style of this book is not prescriptive; it aims to raise awareness of the issues involved in the choice of a particular health education strategy, allowing individual practitioners to decide on their own particular approach. As *Health of the Nation* essentially limits practitioners to the behaviour change model, it is important to try and widen the discussion. Other models of health education do not easily incorporate the strategy as they use different processes and aim for different health goals. However, it is worth considering adapting the strategy to fit a self-empowerment, social change and community development approach to see the issues from a different perspective. Using a different approach may not necessarily achieve the targets aimed for by the White Paper, but in some ways it may be more likely to promote the health of the individual.

The strategy as a behaviour change approach

Practitioners are likely to involve themselves in:

- the identification of risky behaviours
- the provision of information

The identification of risky behaviours

One of the central threads running through the*Health of the Nation* is the belief that individuals will enjoy health if they avoid certain risky behaviours. The term 'risk' implies that there is a possibility that the behaviour may lead to some form of negative health outcome. However, for some behaviours this negative health outcome may be more of a probability.

These risky behaviours include:

- active or passive smoking
- eating a diet high in salt, fats and sugar
- lack of physical activity
- excessive alcohol consumption
- sunbathing without protection
- having multiple sexual partners
- having unprotected sex
- failing to wear a seatbelt
- reckless driving

Likewise, risk factors identify certain factors that are considered to be associated with higher incidences of disease. The extent to which the individual has any risk factors determines his susceptibility to the disease. These risk factors are used to account for the fact that some individuals develop a disease while others do not.

Examples of risk factors:

- ethnicity
- gender
- familial tendencies

- psychosocial factors; eg. stress and unemployment
- socio-economic group
- obesity
- diabetes
- skin type

It is worth noting that individuals will be powerless to do anything about the presence of many of these risk factors, eg. diabetes. In addition, some clients will be unable to change their risky behaviours because these behaviours fall outside their sphere of influence; for example, the opportunity of attending a regular exercise class is beyond the means of many individuals.

The following should also be considered:

- the majority of people take risks as part of their everyday life (however small these risks may be)
- the presence of a risk factor or a risky behaviour does not guarantee the incidence or the severity of the disease; they only offer information as to the relative risk
- the individual may be aware of the health risks of his behaviour
- diseases and illnesses cannot be attributed to isolated risk factors. There is a more complex picture to consider. A person is the product of his individual experience and his social, physical and cultural environment

It is also important to note that the causal significance (in other words, the strength of the link between the risk factor/behaviour and the incidence rate of the disease) of these risk factors/behaviours is constantly being researched; what is accepted as fact today may be superseded by new findings tomorrow. This process may cast doubts in the eyes of the public on the validity of the results.

The provision of information

Health information needs to not only be given to patients and relatives, but also to nurses' own families and friends. This information is likely to include consideration of the following subjects:

- promoting health of the individual
- safe practices
- health risks
- screening tests/treatment issues

Promoting health of the individual:

Examples of professional practices to promote the health of the individual in relation to the*Health of the Nation* key areas include:

- the occupational health nurse running a workshop to raise awareness amongst nurses about the factors that promote mental health at work·
- the sexual health advisor setting up a visual display in a genito-urinary clinic about the positive aspects of sexual health, for example:
  + contribution to the quality of close relationships
  + enjoyment
  + contribution to feelings of self-esteem and self-worth
  + control of fertility
  + motherhood/fatherhood

Safe practices

Similarly, there are various ways that nurses can provide information about safe practices to others:

- the nurse on the paediatric ward can raise a mother's awareness about safety issues in the home
- the occupational health nurse can run a 'safety in the sun' awareness campaign for staff
- the practice nurse can inform women about effective breast examination
- the nurse can inform her partner about safer sex
- the ward nurse can provide information about safe alcohol limits to a patient

- the cardiac rehabilitation nurse can inform a patient about the physical and emotional benefits of exercise

Health risks:

The scope for providing information about health risks is also extensive in the form of:

- the ward nurse offering a leaflet about the side effects of smoking to a relative
- the casualty nurse setting up a display about the local rates and causes of childhood accidents in the accident and emergency department
- posters depicting the health risks of inactivity and obesity
- the school health nurse running a workshop for teenagers to address the risks of over-exposure to the sun
- the health visitor informing a family of the health risks of smoking
- the midwife giving information about risky sexual practices to a woman who is considering the options for contraception

Screening tests/treatment issues:

Raising awareness is not just restricted to informing clients about promoting health, safe practices or considering the potential health risks associated with particular behaviour patterns. It may also involve discussing certain screening tests or treatment issues. The client has a right to weigh up the pros and cons before deciding whether to undergo an operation or test. The following example illustrates this:

- the practice nurse may explain to a woman called for a cervical smear that screening programmes have been shown to effectively reduce both the incidence and mortality of cervical cancer. She explains that as pre-cancerous stages of the disease can be detected, treatment can start early which in turn reduces the number of women that have to go on to have radical surgery. However, the practice nurse also discusses the discomfort of the procedure and informs the woman that some smears are difficult to read accurately

Ways to provide the information

Information may be provided in the following ways:

- in a leaflet
- as a visual display or exhibition
- in a video recording
- during a one-to-one discussion
- during a lecture to a group
- during a workshop or focus group

Personalising the information

The health information needs to be discussed within the context of the individual's social and cultural environment. The social and cultural context of certain health behaviours is apparent when the following issues are considered:

- diet — in some households it may be just one partner who does all the shopping and cooking, thereby controlling to a certain extent what the other partner eats. Work and shift patterns may govern how and when families eat. Certain foods may also have a cultural significance
- weigh —: an individual's appearance may be perceived by others to reflect his inner self. If an individual is considered overweight he may be labelled as lazy or low in self-esteem
- exercise — there are sex differences in participation in physical activity which are influenced by current attitudes about what is suitable for women and men; importantly, exercise is often only regarded as positive and healthy. However, it can also lead to joint and muscle injury
- smoking — smoking may provide a way of coping with the routines of the day. It may be a means of relaxation and pleasure for an individual to enable him to cope with stress and boredom of daily routine
- sunbathing — the presence of a tan is still considered an attraction and a symbol of pleasure, ie. a holiday. The other side of the picture is that excessive exposure to ultraviolet light is also known to lead to premature ageing of the skin

- safer sex — there are various reasons why individuals choose not to use condoms:
  - ✢ it can be embarrassing to buy them
  - ✢ the cost may be prohibitive
  - ✢ it may be difficult to master the technique of application
  - ✢ there may be a fear that the sheath will affect the quality of sexual activity or sensations
  - ✢ sex may lose its spontaneity
  - ✢ there is a certain stigma attached to the idea of carrying condoms about on your person; being in the possession of a supply of condoms can be perceived as a sign of promiscuity
  - ✢ insistence on a change in practice demands social skills and self-confidence which many partners may lack
  - ✢ using a condom necessitates forward planning and concern for health in the long term; however, many sexual encounters are prompted by a need for immediate physical and social gratification
  - ✢ taking the initiative in sex can be hard for women in general as the prevailing culture is still male dominated
- reckless driving — advertising campaigns tend to focus on the fast car as a stereotype of masculinity. The images used are designed to excite and appeal to those who enjoy power and speed, and are willing to take risks

It is important to acknowledge that a proportion of people will choose not to change their lifestyle, despite receiving information on the associated health risks. Even if a nurse personalises her information, some individuals will wish to take this risk and continue with the risky behaviour.

For example, a nurse may encounter a client who openly admits that he is having sex without protection. The nurse is likely to discuss with the client:

- the client's behaviour
- how his sexual behaviour fits into his lifestyle
- reasons for his behaviour
- the client's particular risks associated with the behaviour

The client may consider changing his practice after the discussion. However, even if the client chooses not to adopt safer sexual practices it is important that the nurse demonstrates her acceptance of this choice.

Summary:

- implementation of the *Health of the Nation* strategy within its existing behaviour change framework involves targeting those individuals who have risky lifestyles
- there are a number of risk factors or risky behaviours which identify an individual as being more susceptible to a disease than his colleague; their presence does not however guarantee the incidence or severity of the disease
- nurses may need to not only provide information for individuals about their health risks, but also to discuss the promotion of their health and implementation of safe practices; in addition, treatment issues may need to be considered
- this information can be provided in a variety of ways, e.g. as a leaflet or a talk
- this information needs to be personalised and attention paid to the values of certain behaviours

---

The strategy in the form of a self-empowerment approach

The aim of *Health of the Nation* is to initiate lifestyle change so that fewer individuals suffer or die from diseases, such as cancer or stroke. A self-empowerment model does not easily incorporate this strategy as its success is measured not on a change of behaviour, but on the individual's acquisition of skills which enables him to assume greater control of his health.

Nurses can still use the *Health of the Nation* key areas as a basis to work from, but instead of working from a medically defined model of health they need to work from the individual's own agenda. This move to encompass the client's definition of health is often not easy, as acknowledged in chapter four. However, there is still scope for client empowerment.

The scope for empowerment

For example, a young man is admitted to a coronary care unit with his first attack of chest pain. He is told by his doctor that he must give up smoking and change his diet. The nurses find that he continues to smoke secretly and displays little interest in any of their educational sessions about smoking and diet.

This man is actually terrified that he is going to lose his job as a heavy goods driver. While he feels that he has little control over the incidence and severity of his chest pain, and even less control over events at work, he is unlikely to be able to make important decisions about his health. This feeling of stress exacerbates his need for cigarettes.

Although the nurse is unable to relieve these stressors directly, she can enable the patient to feel that he is able to have some influence over his situation. She can enable him to acknowledge why he feels anxious. She can teach him about angina, allowing him to identify what brings on the attacks and how he can adapt accordingly. The nurse can also put the patient in touch with the relevant social service personnel so that he can work out his options about his future employment.

Once the driver feels that he can influence the outcome of his problems he may then wish to consider whether changing certain behaviours will have a positive effect on his health. If he expresses a desire to alter his smoking pattern, the nurse can help him to identify the following:

- possible triggers for this decision
- particular reasons for him wanting to cut down or stop smoking.

- potential losses and benefits of cessation
- important sociocultural factors that may affect his ability to give up smoking
- his anxieties about giving up the habit
- possible support systems
- possible withdrawal symptoms

Appropriate support may be provided in the form of:

- provision of appropriate literature
- referral to a local smoking cessation group
- involvement of other important family members
- professional follow-up and support

Self-empowerment methods can also be used in the following situations:

- the sexual health advisor enabling an individual to work through his feelings about having HIV and plan ways to cope for the future
- the school nurse facilitating a teenager to come to a decision about his own sexual behaviour by allowing him to express and understand his feelings about his sexuality
- the occupational health nurse working with a staff nurse who is finding it hard to cope in the workplace; the nurse is then able to develop and initiate her own health plan
- the rehabilitation nurse enabling a couple to come to terms and adapt to one partner's disabilities resulting from a stroke
- the midwife providing a woman who is having difficulty adjusting to motherhood with the support and professional guidance required for the mother to overcome her difficulties with breast feeding

Summary:

- adapting *Health of the Nation* so that it fits within a self-empowerment approach involves a shift from adoption of a professional definition of health to one that is defined by the individual
- there is scope for initiatives involving self-empowerment in the key areas

The strategy in the form of a social change approach

The problem with trying to fit the *Health of the Nation* into a social change approach is that the White Paper sets out an individualistic strategy which largely ignores the social and economic determinants of health. The strategy shifts the emphasis onto the individual, but fails to recognise the importance of providing socio-economic support to enable the individual to make his health choices. However, within the key areas are central themes of social and structural disadvantage. These can be used to shape an action framework for health promotion.

Initiating structural changes

Action is likely to take the form of the following strategies:

- raising awareness amongst professional colleagues
- lobbying for local action
- campaigning for wider social changes

Raising awareness among professional colleagues

The politics of health is often a neglected topic in nursing. Part of the way to encourage nurses to adopt a more proactive role in fighting for health for all is to ensure that they are aware of those factors that militate against this goal. One method of doing this is to provide this information for nurses in the form of professional development updates. Political issues such as the influence of the tobacco industry on health and influences on food choices (see below) can be raised to generate discussion.

The influence of the tobacco industry on health:

- by allowing the tobacco industry to continue to promote and sell tobacco, the Government is indirectly acknowledging the value of smoking
- this value is in economic terms because of the revenue received and the employment provided by the sale of tobacco
- a total ban on advertising, restricting smoking in public places and increasing the price of tobacco are likely to be more effective deterrents than the government's existing plan of action
- as smoking rates drop in Europe due to aggressive anti-smoking policies, the tobacco industries are likely to target the developing countries

Influences on food choices:

- the agriculture and food industries combined are the largest industries in the United Kingdom
- due to price initiatives and various forms of government control, the market encourages the production of certain 'unhealthy' foods, such as sugar and fatty meat
- food consumption is affected by access to and availability of healthy foods at affordable prices
- the higher rates of coronary heart disease in the industrial world could be due to the long-term changes in the methods of food advertising, distribution and manufacture
- the new hypermarkets discriminate against the low income groups as they are usually situated out of town and therefore better suited for those with their own transport

Lobbying for local action

Fighting for the provision of a working environment that supports and promotes the health of its staff is important. It may be that various groups representing different causes lobby independently for a healthy working environment. Alternatively, a working party might be formed specifically in order to place health high on the agenda of the organisation.

This may mean fighting for the provision of certain facilities.

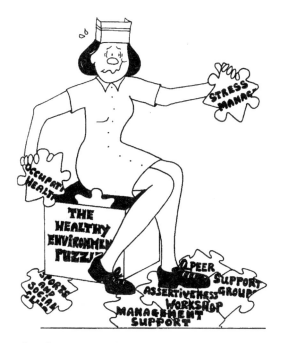

Providing for the mental health of employees:

- supportive management structures
- an organisational culture that recognises achievement and involves staff in decision making
- policies and procedures that support the promotion of health, eg. healthy eating policy, alcohol in the workplace policy
- effective supervision
- stress management workshops

- assertiveness training
- staff support groups
- leisure facilities
- a social club
- access to counselling
- access to forms of relaxation, such as massage therapy, aromatherapy

Providing for the sexual health of employees:

- the provision of courses to enable nurses to have the necessary communication and counselling skills to deal with clients' needs
- free condoms in recreational areas, social clubs
- the provision of HIV/AIDS training courses to raise staff's awareness of the current issues and to encourage nurses to examine their own beliefs and prejudices
- access to a clinical nurse specialist who is responsible for education, changing practice and research
- access to an occupational health service which can offer advice on contraception, needle stick injuries and sexual health

This working party of health-care professionals may lobby their employer to remove the total smoking ban that is operational within their trust. They may agree that it is necessary to restrict smoking to certain areas in order to:

- protect the rights of non-smokers
- assist those who wish to give up
- prevent passive smoking

However, they may consider that a smoking ban can:

- violate the rights of smokers
- restrict the principle of choice manifested in the Patient's Charter
- promote the fallacy that health behaviour is determined by individual choice
- blame the smoker and somehow associate smoking with a sense of moral inadequacy

- encourage secret smoking with an associated risk of fire
- foster the idea that the health professional knows best for the patient

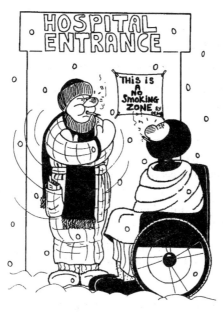

The group may fight for further support for those who want to give up smoking, together with the provision of designated areas which are pleasant and well-ventilated for those who wish to carry on smoking.

Campaigning for wider social changes

Campaigning may not only be directed at local level. Nurses may unite together to fight for wider social and structural changes. This may involve:

- health visitors campaigning to make the wearing of cycle helmets compulsory for children
- mental health nurses uniting to fight for a restriction on the use of benzodiazepines
- nurses campaigning for a ban on tobacco advertising

Summary:

- adapting *Health of the Nation* to fit a social change model necessitates a shift in emphasis away from the individual towards a collective responsibility for health; instead of targeting the individual, attention is focused on the central themes of social and structural disadvantage
- implementation of this approach may involve nurses in raising awareness of the political agenda to health, lobbying for local action and campaigning for wider social issues

The strategy in the form of a community development approach

As acknowledged earlier, the method of empowering people to choose and implement their own health plan does not sit easily within the framework of 'Health of the Nation'. However, group health needs often coincide with some of the themes of ill-health which run through the strategy.

Working with groups

Nurses are likely to work with:

- self-help groups providing support for each other
- client groups fighting for services that are based on the needs of the clients

Both types of group can influence decision making and raise awareness. They can also challenge professional and public attitudes and beliefs.

Self-help groups providing support for each other

For example, family members of individuals with a drug addiction may form a group to provide support for one another. The members may involve health professionals in order to raise the public profile of the purpose of their group. They may also ask certain nurses to provide information for their benefit. A school nurse may be invited to talk about the workshops that she runs to aid the prevention of drug use in teenagers.

Client groups fighting for services that are based on the needs of the clients

In another case a mental health nurse may work with a group of carers in the community who have united to fight for their health needs. The carers have identified that:

- services are often inaccessible for some of the clients with mental health problems
- there is a lack of appropriately translated information for clients and carers
- there is a lack of professional support for carers

The nurse may facilitate the group in its early stages and then withdraw once the group has formed and is making progress. In addition to acting as advocate for the group, the nurse can also provide the following:

- epidemiological information
- names and addresses of relevant health service/social service personnel to lobby
- professional support for the campaign
- resources; a venue for the group to meet, limited funding
- a stand at a local health centre for the group to advertise its message
- social networks of other similar projects

Summary:

- *Health of the Nation* can be incorporated into a community development approach by picking up on those themes of disadvantage and ill-health which are pertinent to the group
- implementation of this approach may involve nurses working with self-help groups or particular client groups providing information, acting as a resource and giving support as

References

Department of Health (1992) *The Health of The Nation: A Strategy for Health in England*. HMSO, London

Department of Health (1993) *Targeting practice: The Contribution of Nurses, Midwives and Health Visitors*. HMSO, London

Further reading

Targeting risky behaviours

King's Fund (1988) *The Nation's Health: A Strategy for the 1990s*. King's Fund, London
● This book provides details of statistical material about health trends

McBride A (1995) *Health Promotion in Hospital: A Practical Handbook for Nurses*. Scutari Press, London
● This book provides knowledge and facts about specific lifestyle issues

McKie L (1994) *Risky Behaviours and Healthy Lifestyles: A practical guide to health promotion*. Quay Books, Dinton, Nr Salisbury
● This book discusses definitions and assessments of risky behaviours

Empowering individuals

Seedhouse D, Cribb A (1989) *Changing Ideas in Health Care*. John Wiley and Sons, Chichester
● This book explores different innovations in health care, all of which uphold the themes of holism, equality and autonomy

Blackburn C, Graham H (1992) *Smoking among Working Class Mothers: Information Pack*. Department of Applied Social Studies, University of Warwick, Warwick
● This is a useful information pack designed to help nurses, midwives and health visitors understand the links between social conditions, motherhood and smoking. The pack also provides pointers for practice

Ewles L, Simnett I (1992) *Promoting Health: A Practical Guide*,
2nd edn. Scutari Press, London
- Chapter 10 provides a useful guide to aid nurses to plan a strategy
  to clarify clients' values and increase their self-awareness

Implementing social change

Ewles L, Simnett I (1992) *Promoting Health: A Practical Guide*,
2nd edn. Scutari Press, London
- Chapter 13 discusses the development and implementation of
  policies. It also considers campaigning

McKie L (1994) *Risky Behaviours and Healthy Lifestyles: A
Practical Guide to Health Promotion*. **Quay Books, Dinton, Nr
Salisbury**
- This book explains about the design and implementation of public
  policies

Working with communities

Ewles L, Simnett I (1992) *Promoting Health: A Practical Guide*,
2nd edn. Scutari Press, London
- Chapter 12 looks at working with communities

McKie L (1994) *Risky Behaviours and Healthy Lifestyles: A
Practical Guide to Health Promotion*. **Quay Books, Dinton, Nr
Salisbury**
- This book discusses the practicalities of community health projects

Wilson J (1992) Ready for take-off. *Nurs Times* **88**(10): 26–8
- This article provides information about the role of the nurse in
  facilitating groups with a view to the formation of self-help groups

Chapter 6

Thoughts for the future

Much of the early discussion in this book has focused on issues surrounding the concept and practice of health promotion. The aim of the book is also to consider the implementation of health education (as part of health promotion) within nursing practice, with special reference to the various initiatives that can be undertaken by nurses working towards achieving the targets under the umbrella strategy, *Health of the Nation* (Department of Health, 1992).

This chapter addresses:

- The changing face of nursing
- The theory–practice gap in health promotion
- A three-point plan to address the divide
- Pointers for practice
- Concluding comments

In chapter four it is acknowledged that humanistic values such as holism, equality and autonomy which are central to nursing are also essential building blocks for the promotion of health. In contrast, it is now apparent that key themes such as enablement, collaboration, mediation and community participation, which together represent the very *essence* of health promotion, do not always sit easily within the realms of nursing practice.

This may not be because the conceptual framework for nursing practice is at odds with that for health promotion practice in nursing. Health education and health promotion are complex subjects and practitioners require certain skills, knowledge, clear strategies and the presence of a supportive environment to translate theory successfully into practice. Often nurses themselves do not share a common understanding of the value and purpose of nursing. It is no surprise then to see that they also share different *wo*rld views' about health promotion.

The purpose of this chapter is to focus on these inconsistencies in the light of the changes currently affecting nursing practice and to suggest a structured way forward for health promotion practice for nurses.

The changing face of nursing

The nursing profession has developed rapidly over the past 15 years. It has had to respond to certain external influences as well as to develop in response to pressures originating from within the profession itself.

External/internal influences on nursing

Societal patterns:
- increasing numbers of elderly
- reduction in the numbers of school leavers
- reduction in the numbers entering nursing

NHS changes:
- increased consumerism
- purchaser/provider status; contracting for services has placed greater emphasis on efficiency and effectiveness
- junior doctors' initiative to reduce the numbers of hours worked
- introduction of resource management

- *Community Care Act* (Department of Health, 1989); *Health of the Nation* (Department of Health, 1992); *The Patient's Charter* (Department of Health, 1991)

Professional initiatives:

- clinical regrading
- increased focus on community development and primary health care
- introduction of Project 2000 and move to higher education
- introduction of health care assistants
- post-registration education and practice (PREP)
- *Scope of Professional Practice* (United Kingdom Central Council for Nursing, Midwifery and Health Visiting, 1992)

Nursing has also been obliged to raise the profile of health promotion within the profession. Over the last 15 years there has been increasing pressure for health promotion theory to be incorporated into nursing practice.

The role of the nurse is likely to come under further scrutiny in the light of current changes in the NHS, in particular:

- to meet the needs of the population
- to change working practices in keeping with other professional groups
- to influence the development of nursing as a profession

Possible future developments in nursing:

- increased focus on bridging boundaries between acute and community-focused care
- greater understanding and use of the role of advocacy; shifting the power balance from professional to client
- development of team-working between professional groups; concentrating on collaborative care and shared goal setting
- definition of outcomes and benchmarks of good-quality nursing practice

- development of a career pathway for clinical nursing practice; definition of the role of the specialist and advanced practitioner with clear guidelines for the educational support required
- establishment of systems of clinical support/direction for practitioners through clinical supervision and reflective practice
- increased emphasis on quality and audit
- increased focus on accountability and new roles (*The Scope of Professional Practice*)

The list above illustrates potential areas of expansion which, if explored, could lead to further excellence in nursing practice. Some of the themes, if developed, would also facilitate the *emancipation* of the nurse's role as a health promoter.

For example, the role of the health visitor is currently under review. If health visiting as a profession develops in order to reflect the needs of the population it serves, then it could become more involved in community projects and initiatives. Instead of working with individuals or families, health visitors could collaborate and work closely with local groups to identify their particular needs. Health visiting could then become instrumental in shaping the purchasing and provision of care to suit the needs of the community.

Summary:

- the face of nursing has changed markedly over the past 15 years in response to external as well as internal pressures
- nursing is likely to continue to develop further in order to meet the needs of the population it serves, to maintain its professionalism and to enhance working relationships with colleagues
- some of the initiatives currently being advocated as important for the growth of nursing as a profession may also facilitate the emancipation of the nurse's role as health promoter

---

The theory–practice gap in health promotion

It is quite clear that although nurses now seem generally more aware of the importance of health promotion in nursing, there is still a large gap between what is advocated to be the way forward and what is actually practised by the majority of nurses. The behaviour change and educational model of health education can be criticised for assuming that there is a straightforward progression from knowledge to attitude change to behaviour change. In reality, people make choices for more complex reasons; just knowing about the benefits about giving up smoking is often not enough to persuade an individual to change his behaviour. Similarly, it is naive to expect that simply raising nurses' awareness of the importance of health promotion will be sufficient to change nursing practice.

So how can change be facilitated within nursing practice? The self-empowerment model relies on the principle that individuals need to internalise the health information they receive so that it assumes a particular meaning for them. Only when the knowledge of the health information has a personal value attached to it, is there the potential for the individuals to actually change their behaviour. In addition, the individuals must then develop certain skills to enable them to act on this information.

So perhaps the reason why nurses have so far struggled and generally failed to incorporate a central focus on promoting health into their practice is because:

- nurses fail to identify with the ideology of health promotion (i.e. nurses generally do not identify themselves with the thoughts and values that underpin health promotion theory)
- nurses often lack the skills required to translate theory into practice

In addition, it has already been noted that, in targeting the health of the individual, the self-empowerment model can be criticised for not directly tackling the existing social, political and environmental injustices. In a similar way then, it can be seen that the third barrier to effective implementation of health promotion relates to the prevailing culture of the nursing profession.

Thus, a strategy for the way forward must incorporate the following:

- an exploration of nurses' world view of health and health promotion; they need to identify those values which are consistent with nursing practice
- recognition among nurses of the skills required to promote health effectively; they must also be committed to a programme for the development of these skills
- recognition among nurses of the impact that rigid demarcations within the profession have on their role; they need to demonstrate a commitment to break entrenched practices

Summary:

- currently there is a large theory–practice gap in health promotion practice in nursing
- this gap has arisen because nurses have failed to internalise the values and beliefs of health promotion theory, they lack the skills required to apply the theory in practice and they belong to a profession which has so far collectively failed to tackle the injustices entrenched within nursing's social context
- the way forward involves enabling nurses to identify with the philosophy of health promotion, allowing nurses to develop their practice skills and facilitating nurses to address the social/cultural/political factors that have influenced the development of the nursing profession

A three-point plan to address the divide

1.   Developing a philosophy of health promotion

Before considering how to enable nurses to identify themselves with the thoughts and values that underpin health promotion theory, it is important to take a step back and examine nurses' identification with the ideology of nursing theory.

Over the last 15 years a lot of interest and attention has focused on models for clinical nursing practice. It was claimed that these models would provide nursing with scientific credibility, facilitate the practice of new ideas and provide nurses with the structure and framework needed to guide their practice. While their value in providing a frame of reference is accepted, it has now been acknowledged that there have been a number of problems involved in their practical application:

- often the choice of model has been imposed on the group of practitioners. A model is based on a philosophy of nursing care; it is constructed around a set of values and beliefs. If nurses are forced to use a particular model, they may not identify with the author's view of nursing. For example, the widespread use of nursing models in midwifery practice has caused problems as midwives perceive their values and beliefs to be different from those of nurses. The majority of nursing models are illness-based, while midwives place emphasis on being health-based.
- often the model has reduced the art of nursing to a series of systems and scientific theories. Some models use long words and complex frameworks which are difficult to translate into practice and difficult to explain to the client. These models do not encourage client participation in care.

Important lessons to be learnt from this:

- models of health education are useful as terms of reference. However, they can oversimplify the issues and lose sight of the spirit of health promotion in its broadest sense

- models of health education practice should not be imposed on practitioners either by managers or educationalists. Practitioners need to examine their own health beliefs and values and then choose a particular model of health education as part of health promotion practice, which reflects their shared philosophy
- models of nursing must be explored to see on what philosophy they are based. Some models focus on illness not health and discourage client and family involvement. It may be difficult to incorporate a health promotion focus into these frameworks

---

Summary:

- models for practice should ideally provide a framework to ensure consistency between what nurses believe and what they do
- the choice of health promotion model for practice should reflect the practitioners' shared philosophy
- The choice of nursing model for practice should also reflect these same values and beliefs

---

Evaluating health education practice

Once nurses have examined their values and beliefs and chosen an approach to health education which reflects these, it is important for them to consider how their methods will be evaluated in practice. Thus their philosophy should be evident in both the implementation of the programme and in the way it is evaluated.

It is important to measure the success of health education practice in the same way that nursing care is evaluated on a continual basis. Formalising the evaluation process has two purposes:

- it focuses nurses' attention on the *process* of health education (ie. did the method reflect the original aim of the exercise?)
- it focuses nurses' attention on the *outcome* of health education (ie. was the aim achieved?)

Evaluation can involve:

- the nurse — measuring her perceptions of her practice
- the client — measuring the effect of the process, the actual outcome and the clients' perceptions of practice

Examples of evaluation methods are included in the table below:

Evaluation methods of behaviour change model	Evaluation methods of educational model	Evaluation methods of self-empowerment model
process: evaluation of attendance cards to see if a client has attended all of his weight reduction classes	*process*: use of a questionnaire or interview to see if a client expresses a positive attitude about the style of teaching he received	*process*: evaluation of a client's diary recording his feelings about his diet
outcome: evaluation of weight charts to see if a client has lost weight	*outcome*: use of a questionnaire to assess a client's increase in knowledge about diet	*outcome*: use of a focus group to assess the change in a client's attitude about his weight

Summary:

- the success of health education practice needs to be evaluated on a regular basis
- the process and outcome of the practice should reflect the philosophy of the health education approach chosen

2.   Developing practice skills

All nurses will have their own definition of the concept of health and health promotion. Their definitions are likely to be based on their world views. Exposing nurses to the knowledge explored by psychologists, sociologists, economists and health promotion specialists may add a different perspective and form a new backdrop to their world views.

Developing a knowledge base for health promotion practice needs to involve the following subjects:

- history of the public health movement
- world patterns of health
- concepts of health including lay health beliefs
- explanations for health behaviour
- cultural/community health patterns
- politics of health
- sociology of health
- theories of health promotion/health education
- alternative styles of learning/teaching
- theories of change management
- healthy public policy
- politics of nursing

However, developing a knowledge base is not sufficient; there are certain skills required for implementation of health promotion theory.

Some of the skills required for health promotion practice:

- advocacy
- empathy
- active listening
- negotiation
- facilitation
- person-centred counselling

- managing change
- campaigning
- lobbying

Some of these practice skills can be gained by attending workshops and courses. Development of these skills is gained by a process of experiential learning. For example, although a nurse may learn about the principles of change management by taking part in a role play, she is unlikely to build up her skills further unless in real life she faces a variety of different situations each of which requires her to adopt a slightly different strategy.

Reflection (in action and on action) is becoming an increasingly important skill in nursing. Nurses are now encouraged to reflect on their practice in order to evaluate the care they give, to question clinical practice and to facilitate change.

Reflection can also be of benefit in developing health promotion practice. It can enable nurses to explore whether the reality of their actions ties in with their professional and personal values and beliefs. In addition, it can facilitate practitioners to identify the wider social and political influences on practice.

Reflection should include consideration of the following influences on health promotion practice:

- ethical factors
- moral factors
- social factors
- political factors

Summary:

- exposure to other disciplines such as psychology and sociology is likely to affect nurses' perceptions about the concept of health and health promotion
- there are a variety of skills required for the effective implementation of health promotion theory
- reflection in action is a useful tool to enable nurses to examine their values and beliefs as evident in practice

3. Developing a supportive professional framework for health

In chapter four attention was drawn to the limitations of the self-empowerment model in practice. It was noted that the culture of an organisation may actually restrict the nurse's practice. In this case it is unrealistic to expect the nurse to empower others when she is not in a position of power herself.

Collectively nurses represent a potentially powerful group. Yet historically they have maintained a low political profile. It is almost as if nurses are *socialised* to assume a quiet, passive stance. Conflict also exists between groups within the profession itself which can be oppressive as well as divisive, preventing nurses uniting to fight for their own health and well-being.

Conflict commonly exists between:
- managers and clinical nurses
- clinical nurses and educationalists
- midwives, health visitors and nurses
- support workers and nurses

Despite the fact that nursing represents a workforce predominantly made up of women, there is frequently little formal recognition of this in the way the profession structures its working practices, shift patterns and child-care facilities. Nurses often express feelings of discontent with their actual role. They also complain of feeling undervalued.

Gender shapes, structures and influences the world of nursing politically, publicly, socially and ethically. Views on nursing are connected to ideas about womanhood. The value of caring is also closely caught up with gender. The concept of caring embraces the role of nurturing and supporting not only on a formal, professional basis, but also in the private domain. The importance of caring in general tends to be marginalised and devalued by the State, and this is represented in the way that caring work is afforded low pay and low status.

The impetus to establish nursing as a profession has been triggered by nurses' desire to raise the status of nursing, as well as to gain credibility, scientific rigour, self-protection and self-regulation. However, the philosophy behind professionalism can also be seen to be at odds with certain values and beliefs about the promotion of health:

- there is a danger that the individuality and creativity of a personal interaction is marginalised in the quest for a scientific foundation to nursing. Caring is more than just a series of tasks; caring involves the forging of a relationship, the quality of which is difficult to measure and reproduce
- the concept of a profession signifies a special body of knowledge. This creates a power base in nursing which limits the channels of communication between patient and nurse
- the concept of a profession involves setting boundaries and recognising the individuality of the nature of nursing; this prevents collaboration and team spirit between different disciplines

Thus, nurses need to value their contributions in maintaining and enhancing the health of others in their present role as carers. Worth needs to be attributed to the role of nurturing and enabling in nursing practice. Preoccupation with professionalism will deny nurses the ability to mediate, collaborate and work in true partnership with clients.

The way forward therefore needs to involve nurses in:

- gaining an understanding of their gendered world of health-care
- working together to establish their value in nursing and health promotion
- fighting collectively for good practice
- establishing themselves as political change agents

Nurses need to:

'challenge the received wisdom that nursing is a maid of all trades, willing to contract and expand an elastic social identity, at the behest of various powerbrokers in the health-care system' (Brown, 1995)

Summary:

- for nurses to successfully promote the health of others, they need to be empowered themselves
- the value of nursing has traditionally been marginalised because of its associations with women's work
- professionalism in nursing may actually serve to devalue what is the essence of quality health promotion
- nurses need to work together to influence the provision and purchasing of health care

---

Pointers for practice

The discussion so far has looked at general principles for the way forward. At this point it will be useful to focus on the three developmental levels of practice outlined by the UKCC as a guide for the development of expertise in nursing (United Kingdom Central Council for Nursing, Midwifery and Health Visiting, 1995). These levels are primary, specialist and advanced practitioner.

A primary practitioner is a qualified nurse at certificate/diploma level (level one or two higher award English National Board; English National Board, 1990). The role of each primary practitioner varies according to their area of practice and their length of experience.

1. The role of the primary practitioner:

- problem solves and manages a caseload of clients
- maintains clinical standards
- supervises practice

Nurse specialists develop from primary practitioners. They are able to demonstrate specialism in areas of clinical practice and provide evidence of skilled leadership, teaching and research.

2. The role of the specialist practitioner:

- acts as patient advocate
- sets clinical standards
- challenges traditional practices
- educates and advises
- tries new innovative approaches
- acts as implementor of change

The third level of practice refers to the role of the advanced practitioner. This nurse is an expert care-giver who possesses advanced skills in clinical practice, leadership, teaching and research.

3. The role of the advanced practitioner:

- adjusts boundaries of nursing practice
- pioneers and develops new roles within nursing
- enables change in nursing practice
- influences policy development
- leads and develops the nursing profession

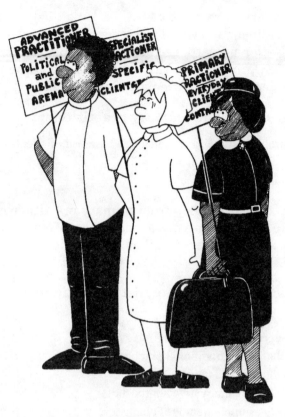

These roles outlined for the primary, specialist and advanced practitioner can be seen to reflect a developmental process involving levels of health promotion practice. For example, while it is unlikely that the primary practitioner has the skills or knowledge to implement a self-empowerment strategy, a specialist practitioner may have the specific skills, be in a position to develop the relationship required and have the power to influence change. Similarly, it may be that only the advanced practitioner is in a position to adopt a political stance for health.

To illustrate this further, Niki Mackintosh has designed a framework outlining the development of particular competencies within health promotion practice, using the

Primary practitioner	Specialist practitioner	Advanced practitioner
Application of practice skills; the ability to:		
• demonstrate communication skills such as empathy and active listening	• demonstrate skills of advocacy, reflection and patient-centred counselling	• demonstrate advanced skills of advocacy, reflection and critical analysis
• demonstrate awareness of role of patient/client advocate	• act as patient/client advocate	• demonstrate skills of effective multidisciplinary team working
• conduct a one-to-one health education session with a patient/client, providing information and raising awareness of health issues	• enable patients/clients to develop certain life skills	• demonstrate skills of effective multi-agency working
• work with groups, providing information and raising awareness of health issues	• facilitate groups, working to their agenda and acting as resource and support	• demonstrate ability to trouble-shoot
Application of health promotional strategies;	*the ability to:*	• demonstrate skills at change management
• demonstrate some awareness of social/ethical/psychological/cultural aspects of health	• demonstrate in-depth knowledge of social/ethical/psychological/cultural aspects of health	• contribute towards the pre- and post- registration education of primary practitioners — **re** social/ethical/psychological/cultural aspects of health **re** approaches to health promotion in practice
• demonstrate an understanding of the different influences on health	• tailor information and adapt methods of health education in recognition of the social/ethical/psychological/cultural needs of the patient/client	• facilitate the provision of a supportive working environment/culture which enables nurses to try new practices

Primary practitioner	Specialist practitioner	Advanced practitioner
(Contd.)		
● demonstrate an understanding of the aims, methods and evaluation of different strategies of health education	● apply the aims, methods and evaluation of different strategies of health education in practice	● demonstrate a pro-active approach in practice
● plan and implement a programme of health education based on the behaviour change/educational model for health education practice	● plan and implement a programme of health education based on the behaviour change/educational/self-empowerment/community development model for health education practice	● plan and implement a programme of health education/promotion based on the community development/social change model set standards for health promotion practice
evaluation methods; the ability to:		
● define outcome measures for behaviour change/educational model for health education practice	● measure outcomes for behaviour change/educational/self-empowerment/community development model for health education practice	● measure outcomes for social change in health promotion practice
management of ethical issues; the ability to:		
● demonstrate awareness of the ethical implications of each of the strategies of health education	● demonstrate in-depth knowledge of the ethical implications of each of the strategies of health education	● contribute towards the pre and post registration education of primary practitioners re ethical implications of health promotion practice

Primary practitioner	Specialist practitioner	Advanced practitioner
(contd.) *influencing policy development; the ability to:* • demonstrate awareness of policy developments *development of research; the ability to:* • demonstrate understanding of research in health promotion • apply health promotion research findings in nursing practice	• contribute towards health policy development • contribute towards a strategy for health promotion for the organisation • disseminate health promotion research findings • initiate change based on health promotion research findings • implement health promotion research	• influence choice of funds for priority areas, using results of needs assessments/health trends • forge links with purchasers • influence policy development • influence strategy for health promotion within organisation • define areas that require research and development in health promotion • implement health promotion research • support others undertaking health promotion research

three levels of practitioner detailed above. This framework is not designed to be prescriptive, but to illustrate the process involved for the primary practitioner to develop into an advanced practitioner in health promotion.

Concluding comments

Summary:

- while all nurses are required to promote health, different practitioners will have varying degrees of experience, knowledge and skills in this field
- the UKCC identifies three levels of clinical practice — primary, specialist and advanced — which can be used as a framework to mark the progress of developing expertise in health promotion in nursing practice

The spirit of health promotion is about enablement, advocacy, mediation and collaboration. It involves not only facilitating people to identify their health needs, but also providing the support they require to implement a health plan and, most importantly of all, providing an environment which allows this process to occur. Health promotion therefore represents a certain set of values, such as holism, equality and autonomy, which influence the attitudes and behaviour of those that practice it. These values are also central to the theory and practice of nursing.

Health promotion is more of a vision for health for all than a certain set of activities. However, different approaches can be adopted to achieve health within this vision. The type of approach adopted will depend on the skills and experience of the nurse as well as the nature of her work. On a busy ward, where emphasis is on speed, partnership in the form of individualised care may be all that is achievable for a primary practitioner. In contrast, a specialist nurse working in the community may be able to expand her role and act as advocate, setting up links between different agencies.

Individuals can only be expected to take some of the responsibility for their health; society also has a large part to play. In the same way, nurses are only one part of the jigsaw which represents health promotion. However, the contribution they make to the overall picture of health needs to be valued and legitimised. As Campbell writes:

> *'...all good nursing is a form of health promotion. It helps the other person mobilise inner resources to deal with the illness or disability and to find those resources which allow the self to resume control. The question for the nursing profession is whether this quiet and often overlooked form of power can find a voice to be heard that will ensure that health promotion is genuine empowerment of the dispossessed and vulnerable'* (Campbell, 1993).

References:

Brown RA (1995) Education for specialist and advanced practice. *Br J Nurs* **4**(5): 266–8

Campbell AV (1993) The ethics of health education. In: Wilson-Barnett J, Macleod Clark J eds. *Research in Health Promotion and Nursing*. Macmillan Press, Hampshire: 20–8

Department of Health (1989) *Caring for People: Community Care in the Next Decade and Beyond*. HMSO, London

Department of Health (1991) *The Patient's Charter*. HMSO, London

Department of Health (1992) *The Health of The Nation: A Strategy for Health in England*. HMSO, London

English National Board (1990) *Framework for Continuing Professional Education and Training for Nurses, Midwives and Health Visitors*. Project Paper 3. ENB, London

United Kingdom Central Council for Nursing, Midwifery and
Health Visiting (1992) *The Scope of Professional Practice*.
UKCC, London

United Kingdom Central Council for Nursing, Midwifery and
Health Visiting (1995) *PREP And You*. UKCC, London

Further reading

Developing a philosophy of health promotion

Caraher M (1995) Nursing and health education: victim blaming.
Br J Nurs **4**(20): 1190–213
- This article explores ideologies and values underpinning health
  education practice. It uses a drama triangle to illustrate types of
  practice that contribute to a healthy relationship

Kitson A (1993) Formalising concepts related to nursing and
caring. In: Kitson A, ed. *Nursing: Art and Science*. Chapman
and Hall, London: 25–47
- This chapter discusses how nurses' perceptions of caring and
  nursing affect their interactions with patients

Lask S, Smith P, Masterson A (1994) *A Curricular Review of the
Pre- and Post-Registration Education Programme for Nurses,
Midwives and Health Visitors in Relation to the Integration of
a Philosophy of Health: Developing a Model for Evaluation*.
ENB, London
- This study found that a philosophy of health had not been
  successfully integrated into pre- and post-registration programmes.
  The authors identified enhancing and hindering factors affecting
  integration of a philosophy of health promotion in the educational
  curricula

Macleod Clark J (1993) From sick nursing to health nursing:
evolution or revolution? In: Wilson-Barnett J, Macleod Clark
J, eds. *Research in Health Promotion and Nursing*. Macmillan
Press, Hampshire: 256–70
- This chapter explores the different philosophy to care embodied in
  sick nursing and health nursing and advocates a move towards the
  latter

Schultz P (1991) Foundations of nursing's perspectives on health
education. *Hoitotiede* **3**(5): 223–30

- This article explores the two practice fields of health promotion and nursing to assess the similarities between the two

Seedhouse D (1988) *Ethics: The Heart of Health Care*. John Wiley and Sons Ltd, London

- This book explores the philosophy of health and provides a detailed theoretical basis for understanding how ethics and health care are interlinked

Wilson-Barnett J (1988) Nursing values: exploring the cliches. *J Adv Nurs* **13**: 790–6

- This article explores the concept of holistic care, individualised care and practical care

Wilson-Barnett J, Latter S (1993) Factors influencing nurses' health education and health promotion practice in acute ward areas. In: Wilson-Barnett J, Macleod Clark J, eds. *Research in Health Promotion and Nursing*. Macmillan Press, Hampshire: 61–71

- This chapter considers the crucial significance of the ward sister in encouraging a certain philosophical approach to care

Developing practice skills

Brown RA, Hawksley B (1996) Learning Skills, Studying Styles and Profiling. Quay Books, Dinton, Wiltshire

Bunton R, MacDonald G, eds (1992) *Health Promotion: Disciplines and Diversity*. Routledge, London and New York

- This book explores the nature of the knowledge base that underpins health promotion

Holland S (1987) Teaching patients and clients — encouraging participation. *Nurs Times* **83**: 59–62

- This article discusses a range of ways to increase patient and client participation

Lask S (1989) Teaching health education. *Nurs Times* **85**(50): 43

- This article describes a course which integrates health promotion concepts into the undergraduate nursing curriculum

Palmer A, Burns S, Bulman C (1994) *Reflective Practice in Nursing: The Growth of the Professional Practitioner*. Blackwell Scientific, Oxford

- This book considers the practice of reflection

Developing a professional framework for health

Campbell AV (1993) The ethics of health education. In:
Wilson-Barnett J, Macleod Clark J, eds. *Research in Health
Promotion and Nursing*. Macmillan Press, Hampshire: 21–8
- This chapter challenges nursing as a profession to break with its
  traditional individualistic approach. Instead he urges it to confront
  the social injustices of health

Davies C (1995) *Gender and the Professional Predicament in
Nursing*. Open University Press, Milton Keynes
- This book examines the implications of gender for the status and
  success of nursing as a profession

Keyzer DM (1988) Challenging role boundaries: conceptual
frameworks for understanding the conflict arising from the
implementation of the nursing process in practice. In: White
R, ed. *Political Issues in Nursing: Past, Present and Future*,
Vol 3. John Wiley and Sons, Chichester: 95–119
- This chapter discusses the difficulties and sources of conflict for
  the clinical nurse working within the new framework for practice

Rose H (1991) Gender politics in the new public health. In:
Draper P, ed. *Health through Public Policy*. Green Print,
London: 159–68
- The author raises gender issues and discusses a way forward for a
  health-promoting environment

Salvage J (1985) *The Politics of Nursing*. Heinemann Nursing,
London
- This book looks critically at nursing and discusses the role of
  politics within the profession

Salvage J (1992) The new nursing: empowering patients or
empowering nurses? In: Robinson J, Gray A, Elkin R, eds.
Policy Issues in Nursing. Open University Press, London:
9–23
- This chapter presents a critical analysis of the role of the new
  practitioner in nursing and explores the social and organisational
  constraints to implementation of patient-centered care

Glossary

Advanced practitioner	A nurse who is an expert care-giver who possesses advanced skills in clinical practice, leadership, teaching and research
Advocacy	Acting on behalf of another, representing another person's cause
Alma Ata	This was a declaration to which the World Health Organization committed in 1977, to improve health for all people by the year 2000
Approach	A particular way of working. Each approach in health education is based upon a model
Behaviour change approach	This approach aims to initiate a change in an individual's lifestyle. Risky behaviours are targeted by the professional
Biomedical approach	This approach focuses on treating illness. Health is perceived as an absence of disease

Community development approach	This approach aims to enable the community to identify and fight for action to meet their health needs
Critical consciousness-raising	Raising awareness of structural and social factors that adversely affect health
Determinism	The belief that individuals are the products of their environments and are therefore not responsible for their health
Educational approach	This approach aims to provide information, but leaves the choice of health action up to the individual
Existentialism	The belief that responsibility for health lies with the individual as he/she has the choice to take a particular health action
Experiential learning	Learning through exposure to certain experiences
Health education	This term refers to the process of transferring knowledge and skills in order to improve understanding and ability
Health promotion	An umbrella term covering a number of measures designed to foster health. Health promotion includes health education and social change
Holism	All parts are essential to the whole
Ideology	The thoughts and values that underpin theory and practice
Lobbying	The process of trying to influence decision making and policy formation

Mediation	Working as an intermediary with different groups to share information, foster relationships and ensure cooperation
Miasma	A term to describe foul air
Model	A set of concepts based upon certain values and beliefs
Multisectoral collaboration	Cooperation and partnership between different agencies and sectors of the population
New public health	Agencies working together in a variety of different ways to achieve a health promoting environment, notably through healthy public policies, campaigning and lobbying
Paternalistic	Protecting the client from harm. Using professional judgment to assess what action is required in the client's best interests
Primary practitioner	A qualified nurse at certificate or diploma level. Different primary practitioners will have varying levels of experience and skill
Public health movement	This term refers to a movement which arose in response to the sudden escalation in disease due to industrialisation in the 1840s. It focused on aspects of the physical environment in its attempt to improve health

Reflection	The process of thinking about an experience, formalising these thoughts, drawing on theory to contextualise the experience and then using this process as a means to develop and learn
Self-empowerment	This approach aims to facilitate the personal development of an individual
Social change approach	This approach aims to address the structural inequalities in health
Specialist practitioner	A nurse with specialist knowledge in an area of clinical practice who also demonstrates skills in teaching, leadership and research
Strategy	Operational outline of a plan for practice
Theory	A set of principles
World view	An individual's perception of or outlook on a subject. This is constructed from his/her knowledge, experience and exposure to certain environments or events

Index